NURSING ASSISTANT/ NURSE AIDE EXAM

NURSING ASSISTANT/ NURSE AIDE EXAM

Fifth Edition

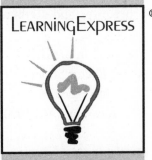

LEARNING EXPRESS ®

NEW YORK

Library of Congress Cataloging-in-Publication Data:
Nursing assistant/nurse aide exam.—5th ed.
        p. ; cm.
    Includes bibliographical references and index.
    ISBN-13: 978-1-57685-895-0
    ISBN-10: 1-57685-895-2
    I. LearningExpress (Organization)
    [DNLM: 1. Nurses' Aides—Examination Questions. WY 18.2]
    610.7306'98—dc23

                                                                        2011043389

Printed in the United States of America

9 8 7 6 5 4 3

Fourth Edition

ISBN 978-1-57685-895-0

Regarding the Information in This Book
We attempt to verify the information presented in our books prior to publication. It is always a good idea, however, to double-check such important information as minimum requirements, application and testing procedures, and deadlines, as such information can change from time to time.

For more information or to place an order, contact LearningExpress at:
    2 Rector Street
    26th Floor
    New York, NY 10006

Or visit us at:
    www.learnatest.com

CONTENTS

LIST OF CONTRIBUTORS ▶

Marlene Beck, RN, MSN is a Nursing Instructor at the Bridgeport Hospital School of Nursing. She has had extensive experience as a manager and educator. In her current position, she has been instrumental in curriculum development, teaching, and clinical supervision. Previously, she was Administrative Manager of Organization, Development, and Education at Bridgeport Hospital/Yale New Haven Healthcare System. In this role, she developed and implemented the first Certified Nursing Assistant program for the hospital. She lives in Seymour, Connecticut.

Patricia Mulrane is a freelance writer with a Bachelor of Arts in Print Media. She began her publishing career in 1994 and is currently Marketing Director for Peter Lang Publishing/USA, a scholarly press in New York City. She lives in Brooklyn, New York.

Mary E. Muscari, PhD, CPNP, APRN-BC started out as a diploma nursing graduate and continued her education to become an advanced practice nurse, educator, and writer. She has written several books and numerous articles, and continues to practice nursing. Dr. Muscari also presents at numerous conferences, inspiring other nurses to find their passions and enhance their careers.

Johanna Rubin, BS, RN works for the New York Harbor HealthCare System as a Compliance Officer, displaying expertise in clinical service education. Her clients include doctors, nurses, and nursing assistants. She is also an instructor at Franklin Career Institute, where she trains beginning nursing assistants.

Caren Silhavey, RN, MSN, CURN is a Nursing Instructor at the Bridgeport Hospital School of Nursing, Bridgeport, Connecticut. Prior to that, she was a Staff Development Instructor in the Organizational Development and Education Department at Bridgeport Hospital, where she taught and coordinated both the Clinical Care Provider program (extended Nursing Assistant) and the Certified Nursing Assistant Program. She lives in Stratford, Connecticut.

National Occupational Competency Testing Institute (NOCTI) is a recognized leader in occupational competency testing and has developed and validated over 250 written exams and performance assessments that measure the skills of entry-level and experienced workers. A non-profit institute, NOCTI has created hundreds of customized workplace-related assessments for major corporations such as Disney, Toyota, GTE, and 3M.

Helen S. Wilson, BSN, RN, is currently an instructor and coordinator of the Certified Nursing Assistant Program at Franklin Career Institute in Hempstead, New York. Previously, she taught the Certified Nursing Assistant programs at Suburban Technical (Hempstead, New York) and Allen School for Nursing Assistants (Queens, New York) and the Licensed Practical Nurse program at VEEB in Uniondale, New York. Before retiring, she served as a Nursing Administrator and Supervisor at the Veterans Affairs Extended Care Facility (Queens, New York). She resides in Uniondale, New York.

NURSING ASSISTANT/
NURSE AIDE EXAM

1 ▶ THE NURSING ASSISTANT/NURSE AIDE EXAM

CHAPTER SUMMARY

This chapter introduces you to the certification process for nursing assistants and shows you how to use this book to help you prepare for the exam to become a Certified Nursing Assistant (CNA).

In this day and age of professionalism, many careers that years ago didn't require much expertise now require not only formal training, but also some type of recognized certification. This trend is particularly true for many healthcare professions, including nursing assistant/nurse aide (NA).

Prior to 1987 there were no standards in nursing homes, and the quality of care was in question. As the public began to hear horrible stories in the media of the abuse and mistreatment of residents in nursing homes, the government decided to step in and take action. The result was the Omnibus Budget Reconciliation Act of 1987 (OBRA '87) that implemented standards for nursing homes that receive federal money, such as Medicare or Medicaid. OBRA '87 also emphasized residents' rights, registered nurse (RN) presence, improved food and medical services for patients, and better maintenance and housekeeping. Due to these new standards, states now individually regulate the training and testing of Certified Nursing Assistants (CNAs).

The information in this book is based on the national standards for CNAs. Because each state specifies the amount of training and what certification and practical-skills exams CNAs must pass, you will also need to contact state or local agencies to find out about the specific requirements in your state.

Finding Out about Certification Requirements

If you want to become a CNA, the first step is to contact your local community or state health agency to obtain certification requirements. You can find these agencies listed in the blue (government) pages of your phone book or by searching online. You can also contact an employment agency or the healthcare facility you want to work for, since they will often be able to guide you through the training and certification requirements. To give you an idea of what to expect, see Chapter 9 for an outline of some of the current trends in CNA certification.

OBRA '87 laws also require that a state registry be kept for CNAs. Information such as dates of certification, reports of abuse and neglect, and lapse periods are available in these registries. Turn to page 4 for a list of registries by state.

Education and Training

Healthcare facilities usually require CNAs to have a high school diploma or GED and pass a state-approved training program that consists of anywhere from 75–150 hours of training. You can be hired without being certified, but you must receive certification within four months. While the duties of a nursing assistant vary depending on the workplace, the job emphasis is always on the physical and emotional well-being of the patient. While a day in the life of a CNA is not easy, especially when dealing with a difficult patient, most get great satisfaction from their work. Common characteristics for someone considering this profession are dedication, patience, reliability, and compassion. Another key element to the job is the ability to communicate and work well with others. A CNA must also be physically able to perform the job, which often requires standing for a good portion of an eight-hour day and lifting and moving objects and equipment. As a CNA, your training will consist of learning to perform the following basic duties:

- communicating with the patient and others on the job
- bathing and dressing the patient (general skin care and hygiene)
- helping patients out of bed
- setting up and storing medical equipment
- taking vital signs—pulse, blood pressure, temperature, and respiration
- feeding the patient
- changing bed linens
- cleaning bedpans and measuring urine output
- answering patient calls and delivering messages

Career Outlook and Earning Potential

The nursing assistant profession, on the whole, is growing faster than average. Nurse aides held about 1.5 million jobs in 2010 and that number is expected to increase by 19% through 2018. While job prospects are good, the salaries tend to be low. Hourly wages range from about $9.23 to $16.45 per hour, depending on which part of the country you live in. Salaries in the Northeast are highest while the South is lower paying. If you have five years of experience or more, your pay increases by a few dollars per hour. Paid holidays, hospital and medical benefits, extra pay for overtime, and pension plans are available to many hospital and some nursing home employees.

Once you know what you have to do to be certified in your state, you can begin to plan your CNA study program. Go to a local job-counseling center, state employment agency, or private healthcare job-placement service to get information about how to get the training you need to become a CNA. Many healthcare agencies will provide you with the training you need. Or you may be able to prepare on your own and simply demonstrate your competence by taking a written exam, a practical exam, or both. Whether you're involved in a training class or working on your own, you should be using textbooks and other materials that will train you in the most important skills a CNA needs. Such books will be available in public libraries and college bookstores; job-search agencies may also have some supplemental materials available.

How to Use this Book

Many state and local agencies require a written exam consisting of approximately 70 multiple-choice questions as part of the certification process for CNAs. This book contains five practice written exams based on the national standards that contain questions about all the skills you will use as a CNA. The written portion of the nursing assistant exam consists of multiple-choice questions, while the clinical portion has the test-taker performing five on-the-job skills. Some of the skills tested include:

- personal care skills, such as client bathing, grooming, dressing, toileting, skin care, and nutrition
- basic nursing skills, such as providing a safe and clean environment, recognizing abnormal signs or symptoms of diseases and conditions, communicating with clients, and understanding basic principles of infection and control
- mental health and social service needs, such as psychosocial characteristics of populations, identification of developmental tasks associated with aging, and behavior management
- basic restorative devices, such as use of assistive devices, range of motion, client transfer, bowel

and bladder training, and care and use of prosthetic devices
- clients' rights, such as privacy, grievances, client and family group participation, physical and chemical restraints, and personal possessions
- employability skills, such as acquiring and maintaining a job

Even if your state or agency doesn't require a written exam, you'll find that these practice exams are a valuable way to review and solidify your skills.

Once you have completed your course of study, you are ready to take the first practice exam in this book. Each practice exam contains 70 multiple-choice questions on all aspects of the job. Allow yourself enough time to complete the entire exam at one sitting, approximately two-and-a-half hours.

Each practice exam has an answer key at the end, which not only tells you the right answer, but also explains why that answer is right. In general, you should count yourself successful when you can score at least 75%. If you don't get that score on the first practice exam, don't panic! First, review the answer explanations to see where you went wrong. Then, see which areas you did well in and which areas gave you more trouble. Go back to your textbook or other training materials to review your weakest areas. Then take the second practice exam. You should find that your score improves. Continue this process—reviewing, taking a practice exam, more review—until you've completed all five practice exams in this book. That way you'll be well prepared for any state certification exam you may have to take.

Practice with the exams in this book is not a guarantee that you will pass a state certification exam—or get a job as a CNA. But it certainly does bring you closer to those goals than if you had not studied and prepared!

In addition to the practice written exams, this book also includes a sample performance assessment in Chapter 8. This is a sample of the kind of job tasks you will perform as a CNA. You may be asked to perform tasks like these either during a state certification exam or by a prospective employer during a job interview. You should practice these tasks and become proficient enough to perform them under pressure with an examiner or your potential employer watching you carefully. Carefully practicing these skills will help you sell yourself to your employer and will put you ahead of other people applying for the same position. Keep in mind that the best-trained person is usually the one who is selected for the position.

Here are the steps to take to become a CNA:

1. Contact local employment agencies or the state health office to find out about certification standards. (A list of state registries follows.)
2. Contact local employment agencies for employment opportunities.
3. Take your CNA course, and/or use study guides and textbooks to prepare for certification.
4. Take the first practice exam in this book and score it. Review your weakest areas.
5. Continue to review and take practice exams. Score yourself on each exam to see how prepared you are for the actual certification exam.
6. Once you feel confident, contact your state or local agency to set a date for taking the certification exam.
7. Take the certification exam and pass it!
8. Show prospective employers your certificate. This shows you're ready to start a job and have the initiative to advance once you're hired.

If you faithfully follow these steps, you will be well on your way to a successful career as a certified nursing assistant.

State Nursing Assistant/ Nurse Aide Registries

ALABAMA
Alabama Certified Nurse Aide Registry
The RSA Tower, Ste. 600
201 Monroe St.
Montgomery, AL 36104
Phone: 334-206-5169
Fax: 334-206-5169
Website: https://ph.state.al.us/nurseaideregistry/faq.aspx

ALASKA
Alaska Nurse Aide Registry
Department of Commerce, Community and Economic
    Development
Division of Corporations, Business and Professional
    Licensing
550 W. 7th Ave., Ste. 1500
Anchorage, AK 99501-3567
Phone: 907-269-8169
Fax: 907-269-8196
Website: www.dced.state.ak.us/occ/pnua.htm

ARIZONA
Arizona State Board of Nursing
Nursing Assistant Registration Program
4747 N. 7th St., Ste. 200
Phoenix, AZ 85014-3655
Phone: 602-771-7800
Fax: 602-771-7888
Website: www.azbn.gov

ARKANSAS
Arkansas Nurse Aide Registry
Department of Human Services
Office of Long-Term Care
P.O. Box 8059, Slot S405
Little Rock, AR 72203-8059
Phone: 501-682-6172
Fax: 501-682-8551

CALIFORNIA
Department of Health Care Services
Licensing and Certification Program
CNA/HHA/CHT Certification Unit
P.O. Box 997416, MS 3301
Sacramento, CA 95899-7377
Phone: 916-327-2445
Fax: 916-552-8785
Website: www.cdph.ca.gov/programs/LnC

COLORADO
Colorado State Board of Nursing
1560 Broadway, Ste. 1350
Denver, CO 80202
Phone: 303-894-2430
Fax: 303-894-2821
Website: www.dora.state.co.us/nursing

CONNECTICUT
Connecticut Department of Public Health
410 Capitol Ave., MS# 12 MQA
P.O. Box 340308
Hartford, CT 06134-0308
Phone: 860-509-7603
Fax: 860-509-7286
Website: www.ct.gov/dph

DELAWARE
Division of Long-Term Care Residents Protection
3 Mill Rd., Ste. 308
Wilmington, DE 19806
Phone: 302-577-6661
Fax: 302-577-6672
Website: www.dhss.delaware.gov/dltcrp/cnareg.html

DISTRICT OF COLUMBIA
District of Columbia Board of Nursing
Department of Health
Health Professional Licensing Administration
899 N. Capital St. NE
First Fl.
Washington, D.C. 20002
Phone: 1-877-672-2174
Fax: 202-727-8471
Website: www.hpla.doh.dc.gov

FLORIDA
Department of Health
Certified Nursing Assistants Council
4052 Bald Cypress Way
Bin # C-13
Tallahassee, FL 32399-3251
CNA Registry Line: 850-488-0595
Fax: 850-412-2207
Website: www.doh.state.fl.us/mqa/cna

GEORGIA
Georgia Health Partnership
P.O. Box 105753
Atlanta, GA 30348
Phone: 678-527-3010
Toll-Free: 800-414-4358
Fax: 678-527-3034
Website: www.mmis.georgia.gov

HAWAII
Department of Commerce and Consumer Affairs
Professional and Vocational Licensing Division
P.O. Box 3469
Honolulu, HI 96801
Phone: 808-586-2695
Fax: 808-586-2689
Website: www.hawaii.gov/dcca/pvl/boards/nursing

IDAHO
Idaho Nurse Aide Registry
Division of Medicaid
Department of Health and Welfare
P.O. Box 83720
Boise, ID 83720-0036
Phone: 208-334-6620
Fax: 208-334-3262
Online Search Form: https://registry.prometric.com/registry/publicID

ILLINOIS
Health Care Worker Registry
525 W. Jefferson St., 4th Fl.
Springfield, IL 62761
Phone: 217-785-5133
Fax: 217-524-0137
Website: www.idph.state.il.us/nar

INDIANA
State Department of Health
Division of Long Term Care
2 N. Meridian St., 4B
Indianapolis, IN 46204-3006
Phone: 317-233-7442
Fax: 317-233-7750
Website: www.in.gov/isdh/23260.htm

IOWA
Department of Inspections and Appeals
Health Facilities Division
Lucas State Office Building
321 East 12th St., 3rd Fl.
Des Moines, IA 50319-0083
Phone: 515-281-4077
Toll-Free (in-state only): 866-876-1997
Fax: 515-281-6259
Website: www.dia-hfd.state.ia.us

KANSAS
Health Occupations Credentialing
1000 S.W. Jackson St., Ste. 200
Topeka, KS 66612-1365
Phone: 785-296-6877
Fax: 785-296-3075
Website: www.ksnurseaidregistry.org

KENTUCKY
Kentucky Board of Nursing
312 Whittington Prkwy., Ste. 300
Louisville, KY 40222-5172
Phone: 502-429-3300
Fax: 502-429-3311
Website: www.kbn.ky.gov

LOUISIANA
Louisiana Nurse Aide Registry
5647 Superior Dr.
Baton Rouge, LA 70808
Phone: 225-295-8575
Fax: 225-295-8578
Website: www.labenfa.com

MAINE
Maine Registry of Certified Nursing Assistants
Maine Department of Health and Human Services
State House Station #11
41 Anthony Ave.
Augusta, ME 04333
Phone: 207-624-7300
Fax: 207-287-9325
Website: gateway.maine.gov/cnaregistry

MARYLAND
Maryland Nurse Aide Registry
4140 Patterson Ave.
Baltimore, MD 21215-2254
Phone: 410-585-1990
Fax: 410-764-8042
Website: www.mbon.org

MASSACHUSETTS
Massachusetts Nurse Aide Registry
Department of Public Health
Division of Health Care Quality
99 Chauncy St., 2nd Fl.
Boston, MA 02111
Phone: 617-753-8143
Fax: 617-753-7320
Website: www.mass.gov/eohhs/gov/departments/dph/
programs/nurse-aide-registry.html

MICHIGAN
Michigan Department of Community Health
Bureau of Health Professionals
P.O. Box 30670
Lansing, MI 48909-8170
Phone: 517-335-0918
Fax: 517-241-2895
Website: www.michigan.gov/healthlicense

MINNESOTA
Division of Compliance Monitoring
Nursing Assistant Registry
P.O. Box 64501
St. Paul, MN 55164-0501
Phone: 651-215-8705
In-State Only: 800-397-6124
Fax: 651-215-9697
Website: www.health.state.mn.us/divs/fpc/profinfo/
narinfo/aboutnar.html

MISSISSIPPI
Bureau of Health Facilities—Licensure and Certification
P.O. Box 1700
Jackson, MS 39215-1700
Phone: 601-364-1100
Fax: 601-364-5055
Website: www.msdh.state.ms.us

MISSOURI
Missouri Department of Health and Senior Services
912 Wildwood
P.O. Box 570
Jefferson City, MO 65102-0570
Phone: 573-526-5686
Fax: 573-526-7656
Website: www.dhss.mo.gov/CNARegistry

MONTANA
Department of Public Health and Human Services
2401 Colonial Dr., 2nd Fl.
P.O. Box 202953
Helena, MT 59620-2953
Phone: 406-444-4980
Fax: 406-444-3456
Website: www.dphhs.mt.gov/cna

NEBRASKA
Nebraska Health and Human Service System
Division of Public Health, Licensure Unit Office of Nursing
    and Nursing Support
P.O. Box 95026
Lincoln, NE 68509-5026
Phone: 402-471-3121
Website: dhhs.ne.gov/publichealth/Pages/lis_lisindex.aspx

NEVADA
Bureau of Health Care Quality and Compliance
727 Fairview Dr., Ste. E
Carson City, NV 89701
Phone: 775-684-1030
Fax: 775-684-1073
Website: www.health.nv.gov/hcqc.htm

NEW HAMPSHIRE
New Hampshire Board of Nursing
21 S. Fruit St., Ste. 16
Concord, NH 03301-2431
Phone: 603-271-6282
Fax: 603-271-6605
Website: www.state.nh.us/nursing

NEW JERSEY
New Jersey Department of Health and Senior Services Office of Program Compliance—Nurse Aide Registry
Division of Health Facilities Evaluation and Licensing
P.O. Box 360
Trenton, NJ 08625-0360
Phone: 866-561-5914 or 609-633-9051
Fax: 609-341-3552
Website: www.state.nj.us/health/healthfacilities/index.shtml

NEW MEXICO
DOH/DHI/Health Facility Licensing and Certification Bureau
2040 S. Pacheco St., 2nd Fl., Rm. 413
Santa Fe, NM 87505
Phone: 505-476-9040
Automated Voice System: 505-827-1453
Fax: 505-476-9026
Website: https://dhi.health.state.nm.us/nar/nar.php

NEW YORK
New York State Department of Health
875 Central Ave.
Albany, NY 12206
Phone: 518-408-1297
CNA Verifications Only: 800-918-8818
Website: www.health.ny.gov/health_care/consumer_
information/nurse_aide_registry

NORTH CAROLINA
North Carolina Department of Health and Human Services
Division of Health Service Regulation
Health Care Personnel Registry Section
2719 Mail Service Center
Raleigh, NC 27699-2719
Phone: 919-855-3969
24-Hour Automated Line: 919-715-0562
Fax: 919-733-9764
Website: www.ncnar.org

NORTH DAKOTA
North Dakota Department of Health
Division of Health Facilities
600 E. Boulevard Ave., Dept. 301
Bismarck, ND 58505-0200
Phone: 701-328-2353
Fax: 701-328-1890
Website: https://www.ndhealth.gov/hf/registry/inquiry
-search.aspx

OHIO
Bureau of Information and Operational Support
Ohio Department of Health
Nurse Aide Registry
246 N. High St.
Columbus, OH 43215-2412
In-State Only (automated system): 800-582-5908
Outside Ohio (automated system): 614-752-9500
Fax: 614-564-2461
Website: www.odh.ohio.gov/odhprograms/io/nurseaide/
nurseaide1.aspx

OKLAHOMA
State Department of Health
Nurse Aide Registry
1000 N.E. 10th St., Room 1111
Oklahoma City, OK 73117-1299
Phone: 405-271-4085
Fax: 405-271-1130
Website: www.ok.gov/health/Protective_Health/
Health_Resources_Development_Service/Nurse_Aide_
and_Nontechnical_Services_Workers_Registry/index.html

OREGON
Oregon State Board of Nursing
17938 S.W. Upper Boones Ferry Rd.
Portland, OR 97224-7012
Phone: 971-673-0685
Fax: 971-673-0684
Website: www.oregon.gov/OSBN

PENNSYLVANIA
Pearson VUE/Nurse Aide Registry
P.O. Box 13785
Philadelphia, PA 19101-3785
Toll-Free: 800-852-0518
Website: www.portal.state.pa.us/portal/server.pt/
community/nurse_aide_registry/14154

RHODE ISLAND
Rhode Island Department of Health
Office of Health Professionals Regulation
3 Capitol Hill #105
Providence, RI 02908
Phone: 401-222-5888
Fax: 401-222-3352
Website: www.health.ri.gov

SOUTH CAROLINA
Pearson VUE
P.O. Box 13785
Philadelphia, PA 19101-3785
Toll-Free: 800-852-0518

SOUTH DAKOTA
Board of Nursing
Nurse Aide Section
4305 S. Louise Ave., Ste. 201
Sioux Falls, SD 57106-3115
Phone: 605-362-2760
Fax: 605-362-2768
Website: doh.sd.gov/boards/nursing

TENNESSEE
State of Tennessee Department of Health
Nurse Aide Registry
227 French Landing, Ste. 501
Heritage Place, Metrocenter
Nashville, TN 37243
Phone: 615-532-5171
Toll-Free: 800-778-4504
Fax: 615-248-3601
Website: health.state.tn.us/hcf/nurseaide.htm

TEXAS
NFA Licensing
Department of Aging and Disability Services
P.O. Box 149030
Austin, TX 78714-9030
Phone: 512-438-2050
Toll-Free: 800-452-3934
Fax: 512-438-2051
Website: www.dads.state.tx.us/providers/NF/credentialing

UTAH
Utah Nursing Assistant Registry
550 E. 300 South
Kaysville, UT 84037
Phone: 801-547-9947
Website: www.utahcna.com

VERMONT
Vermont State Board of Nursing
Office of Professional Regulation
National Life Building, North Fl. 2
Montpelier, VT 05620-3402
Phone: 802-828-1505 or 802-828-2396
Fax: 802-828-2484
Website: www.vtprofessionals.org

VIRGINIA
Virginia Board of Nursing
Nurse Aide Registry
9960 Mayland Dr., Ste. 300
Henrico, VA 23233-1463
Phone: 804-367-4569
Fax: 804-527-4455
Website: www.dhp.virginia.gov/nursing

VIRGIN ISLANDS
Virgin Islands Board of Nurse Licensure
P.O. Box 304247, Veterans Dr. Sta.
St. Thomas, VI 00803
Phone: 1-340-776-7397
Fax: 1-340-777-4003

WASHINGTON
DSHS Aging and Adult Services Administration
OBRA Nursing Assistant Registry
P.O. Box 45600
Olympia, WA 98504-5600
Phone: 360-725-2597
Fax: 360-493-2581
Website: www.aasa.dshs.wa.gov/professional/nat

WEST VIRGINIA
Office of Health Facility
Licensure and Certification
408 Leon Sullivan Way
Charleston, WV 25301-1713
Phone: 304-558-0050
Fax: 304-558-1442
Website: www.wvdhhr.org/ohflac/NA

WISCONSIN
Wisconsin Department of Health Services
Division of Quality Assurance
1 W. Wilson St.
Madison, WI 53703
Phone: 608-261-8319
Fax: 608-264-6340
Website: www.dhs.wisconsin.gov/caregiver/NATD/
NATDintro.htm

WYOMING
Wyoming State Board of Nursing
1810 Pioneer Ave.
Cheyenne, WY 82002
Phone: 307-777-7601
Fax: 307-777-3519
Website: www.health.wyo.gov/ohls/CNA.html

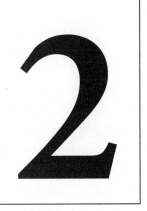

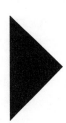

C H A P T E R

THE LEARNINGEXPRESS TEST PREPARATION SYSTEM

CHAPTER SUMMARY

Taking a nursing assistant certification exam can be tough, and your career in healthcare depends on your passing the exam. The LearningExpress Test Preparation System, developed exclusively for LearningExpress by leading test experts, gives you the discipline and attitude you need to succeed.

Passing the CNA certification exam is a rite of passage to your new career, and it allows you to use the CNA credential after your name. Passing may mean more job security and a better salary, and it may be the boost to inspire you to further your nursing career.

Like all good things, passing the exam does not come easily. You do have to work for it. But you don't have to work alone. The LearningExpress Test Preparation System is here to help. In just ten easy-to-follow steps, you will learn everything you need to prepare for the exam and help you perform your best. You'll be in control. Being a "good test-taker" requires more than just knowing your material. It means being prepared.

Here is how the LearningExpress Test Preparation System works: Ten easy steps lead you through everything you need to know and do to get ready to master your exam. Each step includes both reading about the step and one or more activities. It is important that you do the activities along with the reading, or you won't be getting the full benefit of the system.

Step 1: Know the Potential Test-Taking Blockers
Step 2: Get Information
Step 3: Conquer Test Anxiety
Step 4: Make a Plan
Step 5: Learn to Manage Your Time
Step 6: Learn to Use the Process of Elimination
Step 7: Know When to Guess
Step 8: Reach Your Peak Performance Zone
Step 9: Get Your Act Together
Step 10: Do it!

If you have several hours, you can work through the whole LearningExpress Test Preparation System in one sitting. Otherwise, you can break it up and do just one or two steps a day for the next several days. It is up to you—remember, you are in control.

Step 1: Know the Potential Test-Taking Blockers

Activities: Think about tests you had difficulty with in the past. Then take a look at the list of test-taking blockers and see how many of them applied to you back then. Now make your own list from the suggestions for correcting them, place it on your desk or refrigerator, and start making changes.
For example, if you are a negative thinker, write, "Think Positive: I WILL pass my certification exam!"

Part A: Test-Taking Blockers
Test taking is challenging because of the many pitfalls that can keep you from doing your best.

- Having a negative attitude: Thinking that you will do poorly can actually cause you to fail. Think positive. Stand in front of a mirror and say, "I will pass my nursing assistant certification exam!" Post signs around your home and car that say, "I WILL pass!" Write your name with the letters CNA after it.

- Not taking ownership of your career: Teachers don't fail students; students fail on their own. Take ownership of your career. While others may help you, it ultimately remains up to you to pass the certification exam.

- Not preparing for the exam: Don't be overconfident. Even straight-A students can fail exams if they have not prepared.

- Preparing at the last minute: Everyone is pressed for time these days, but you need to make adequate time to prepare for your exam. Weeks are better than days, and days are better than hours. Squeezing several weeks of studying into one night only increases test anxiety. Save that last night for a quick review and a good night's sleep.

- Not practicing: The more you practice nursing assistant exam questions, the better you'll be at answering the ones on your certification exam. Use and reuse the practice exams in this book. You will increase your comfort level and keep getting better at answering multiple-choice questions and performing job-related tasks.

Step 2: Get Information

Activities: Read Chapter 1, "The Nursing Assistant Exam," and use the suggestions there to find out about your certification requirements.
Knowledge is power. Therefore, first, you have to find out everything you can about the nursing assistant exam. Once you have your information, the next steps will show you what to do with it.

Part A: Straight Talk about the Nursing Assistant Exam
Why do you have to take this exam? One of the major objectives of OBRA was to better the quality of care given to residents of long-term care facilities. Thus, OBRA requires that all nursing assistants who wish to work in a long-term care facility complete a training program and pass an exam to ensure they have the

necessary knowledge and skills to provide adequate care. Individual states may or may not require certification to work in acute care facilities (such as hospitals), so you need to check your state's requirements before embarking on the certification process.

It is important for you to remember that your score on the written exam does not determine how smart you are or even whether you will make a good nursing assistant. There are all kinds of things a written exam like this can't test: whether you are likely to show up late or call in sick a lot, whether you can be patient with a trying client, or whether you can be trusted with confidential information about people's health. Those kinds of things are hard to evaluate on a written exam. Meanwhile, it is easy to evaluate whether you can correctly answer questions about the job duties of a nurse aide.

This is not to say that correctly answering the questions on the written exam is not important! The knowledge tested on the exam is knowledge you will need to do your job, and your ability to enter the profession you have trained for depends on your passing this exam. And that's why you are here—to achieve control over the exam.

Part B: What's on the Test

The certification exam tests the skills, knowledge, and attitudes needed to perform as a nursing assistant. These areas include communications, client rights, legal and ethical issues, the healthcare team, grooming and dressing, hygiene, hydration and nutrition, elimination, comfort, rest and sleep, infection control and handwashing, safety, emergencies, therapeutic and technical procedures, data collection and reporting, prevention, self-care and independence, mental health and emotional needs, and spiritual and cultural needs.

The passing score varies by state, but the range is usually from 70 to 80 percent on the written exam. The acceptable score on the clinical skills portion of the exam also varies by state from 70 to 100 percent. Check with your state agency to obtain information about its specific requirements.

Step 3: Conquer Test Anxiety

Activity: Take the Test Anxiety Quiz on page 14.
Having complete information about the exam is the first step in getting control of the exam. Next, you have to overcome one of the biggest obstacles to test success: test anxiety. Test anxiety can not only impair your performance on the exam itself; it can even keep you from preparing! In this step, you will learn stress management techniques that will help you succeed on your exam. Learn these strategies now, and practice them as you complete the exams in this book so that they will be second nature to you by exam day.

Combating Test Anxiety

The first thing you need to know is that a little test anxiety is a good thing. Everyone gets nervous before a big exam, and if that nervousness motivates you to prepare thoroughly, so much the better. Many well-known people throughout history have experienced anxiety or nervousness—from performers such as actor Sir Laurence Olivier and singer Aretha Franklin to writers such as Charlotte Brontë and Alfred, Lord Tennyson. In fact, anxiety probably gave them a little extra edge—just the kind of edge you need to do well, whether on a stage or in an examination room.

Stop here and complete the Test Anxiety Quiz on page 14 to find out whether your level of test anxiety is something you should worry about.

Stress Management before the Test

If you feel your level of anxiety rising in the weeks before the test, here is what you need to do to bring the level down again:

- **Get prepared.** There's nothing like knowing what to expect and being prepared for it to put you in control of test anxiety. That's why you are reading this book. Use it faithfully, and remind yourself that you are better prepared than most of the people taking the test.

TEST ANXIETY QUIZ

You need to worry about test anxiety only if it is extreme enough to impair your performance. The following questionnaire will provide a diagnosis of your level of test anxiety. In the blank before each statement, write the number that most accurately describes your experience.

0 = Never
1 = Once or twice
2 = Sometimes
3 = Often

___I have gotten so nervous before an exam that I simply put down the books and didn't study for it.
___I have experienced disabling physical symptoms such as vomiting and severe headaches because I was nervous about an exam.
___I have simply not showed up for an exam because I was scared to take it.
___I have experienced dizziness and disorientation while taking an exam.
___I have had trouble filling in the little circles because my hands were shaking too hard.
___I have failed an exam because I was too nervous to complete it.
___**Total: Add up the numbers in the blanks above.**

Your Test Stress Score

Here are the steps you should take, depending on your score. If you scored:

- **Below 3**, your level of test anxiety is nothing to worry about; it's probably just enough to give you that little extra edge.

- **Between 3 and 6**, your test anxiety may be enough to impair your performance, and you should practice the stress management techniques in this section to try to bring your test anxiety down to manageable levels.

- **Above 6**, your level of test anxiety is a serious concern. In addition to practicing the stress management techniques listed in this section, you may want to seek additional, personal help. Call your local high school or community college and ask for the academic counselor. Tell the counselor that you have a level of test anxiety that sometimes keeps you from being able to take the exam. The counselor may be willing to help you or may suggest someone else you should talk to.

- **Practice self-confidence.** A positive attitude is a great way to combat test anxiety. This is no time to be humble or shy. Stand in front of the mirror and say to your reflection, "I'm prepared. I'm full of self-confidence. I'm going to ace this test. I know I can do it." If you hear it often enough, you will come to believe it.
- **Fight negative messages.** Every time someone starts telling you how hard the exam is or how it is almost impossible to get a high score, start telling them your self-confidence messages. If the someone with the negative messages is you, telling yourself you don't do well on exams or you just can't do this, don't listen.
- **Visualize.** Imagine yourself reporting for duty on your first day as a certified nursing assistant. Think of yourself helping patients and making them more comfortable. Imagine coming home with your first paycheck. Visualizing success can help make it happen—and it reminds you of why you are working so hard to pass the exam.
- **Exercise.** Physical activity helps calm down your body and focus your mind. Besides, being in good physical shape can actually help you do well on the exam. Go for a run, lift weights, go swimming—and do it regularly.

Stress Management on Test Day

There are several ways you can bring down your level of test anxiety on test day. They will work best if you practice them in the weeks before the test, so you know which ones work best for you.

- **Deep breathing.** Take a deep breath while you count to five. Hold it for a count of one, then let it out for a count of five. Repeat several times.
- **Move your body.** Try rolling your head in a circle. Rotate your shoulders. Shake your hands from the wrist. Many people find these movements very relaxing.

- **Visualize again.** Think of the place where you are most relaxed: lying on the beach in the sun, walking through the park, or whatever makes you feel good. Now close your eyes and imagine you are actually there. If you practice in advance, you will find that you only need a few seconds of this exercise to experience a significant increase in your sense of well-being.

When anxiety threatens to overwhelm you right there during the exam, there are still things you can do to manage the stress level.

- **Repeat your self-confidence messages.** You should have them memorized by now. Say them silently to yourself, and believe them!
- **Visualize one more time.** This time, visualize yourself moving smoothly and quickly through the test answering every question correctly and finishing just before time is up. Like most visualization techniques, this one works best if you have practiced it ahead of time.
- **Find an easy question.** Skim over the test until you find an easy question, and answer it. Getting even one circle filled in gets you into the test-taking groove.
- **Take a mental break.** Everyone loses concentration once in a while during a long test. It is normal, so you shouldn't worry about it. Instead, accept what has happened. Say to yourself, "Hey, I lost it there for a minute. My brain is taking a break." Put down your pencil, close your eyes, and do some deep breathing for a few seconds. Then you will be ready to go back to work.

Try these techniques ahead of time, and see if they work for you!

Step 4: Make a Plan

Activity: Construct a study plan.

Maybe the most important thing you can do to get control of yourself and your exam is to make a study plan. Too many people fail to prepare simply because they fail to plan. Spending hours poring over sample test questions the day before the exam not only raises your level of test anxiety, but also will not replace careful preparation and practice over time.

Don't fall into the cram trap. Take control of your preparation time by mapping out a study schedule. On pages 17 and 18 are two sample schedules, based on the amount of time you have before you take the written exam. If you are the kind of person who needs deadlines and assignments to motivate you for a project, here they are. If you are the kind of person who doesn't like to follow other people's plans, you can use the suggested schedules to construct your own.

Even more important than making a plan is making a commitment. You can't review everything you learned in your nursing assistant course in one night. You need to set aside some time every day for study and practice. Try for at least 20 minutes a day. Twenty minutes daily will do you much more good than two hours on Saturday—divide your test preparation into smaller pieces of the larger work. In addition, making study notes, creating visual aids, and memorizing can be quite useful as you prepare. Each time you begin to study, quickly review your last lesson. This act will help you retain all you have learned and help you assess whether you are studying effectively. You may realize you are not remembering some of the material you studied earlier. Approximately one week before your exam, try to determine the areas that are still most difficult for you.

Don't put off your study until the day before the exam. Start now. A few minutes a day, with half an hour or more on weekends, can make a big difference in your score.

Schedule A: The 30-Day Plan

If you have at least a month before you take the nursing assistant exam, you have plenty of time to prepare—as long as you don't waste it! If you have less than a month, turn to Schedule B.

TIME	PREPARATION
Days 1–3	Skim over a textbook or the written materials from your training program, particularly noting any areas you expect to be emphasized on the exam or any areas you don't remember well.
Day 4	Take the first practice exam in Chapter 3.
Day 5	Score the first practice exam. Based on this exam, identify your strongest and weakest areas. Pick two areas that you will concentrate on before you take the second practice exam.
Days 6–8	Study the two areas you identified as your weak points. Don't worry about the other areas.
Days 9–10	Take the second practice exam in Chapter 4.
Day 11	Score the second practice exam. Identify one area to concentrate on before you take the third practice exam.
Days 12–16	Study the one area you identified for review. In addition, review both practice exams you have taken so far, with special attention to the answer explanations.
Day 17	Take the third practice exam.
Day 18	Once again, identify one area to review, based on your score on the third practice exam.
Days 19–20	Study the one area you identified for review.
Days 21–23	Take an overview of all your training materials, consolidating your strengths and improving on your weaknesses.
Days 24–25	Review all the areas that have given you the most trouble in the three practice exams you have taken so far.
Day 26	Take the fourth practice exam in Chapter 6. Note how much you have improved!
Days 27–28	Review any areas in which you still feel unsure.
Day 29	Take the final practice exam.
Day before the exam	Relax. Do something unrelated to the exam and go to bed at a reasonable hour.

Schedule B: The 10-Day Plan

If you have two weeks or less before you take the exam, you may have your work cut out for you. Use this 10-day schedule to help you make the most of your time.

TIME	PREPARATION
Day 1	Take the first practice exam in Chapter 3 and score it using the answer key at the end. Identify which skill areas need the most work, based on your exam score.
Day 2	Review one area that gave you trouble on the first practice exam.
Day 3	Review another area that gave you trouble on the first practice exam.
Day 4	Take the second practice exam in Chapter 4 and score it.
Day 5	If your score on the second practice exam doesn't show improvement on the two areas you studied, review them. If you did improve in those areas, choose a new weak area to study today.
Day 6	Take the third practice exam in Chapter 5 and score it.
Day 7	Choose your weakest area from the third practice exam to review.
Day 8	Review any areas that you have not yet reviewed in this schedule.
Day 9	Take the fourth practice exam in Chapter 6 and score it.
Day 10	Use your last study day to brush up on any areas that are still giving you trouble and then take the fifth practice exam.
Day before the exam	Relax. Do something unrelated to the exam and go to bed at a reasonable hour.

Learning Styles

Each of us absorbs information differently. Whichever way works best for you is called your dominant learning method. If someone asks you to help them construct a bookcase they just bought that may be in many pieces, how do you begin? Do you need to read the directions and see the diagram? Would you rather hear someone read the directions to you—telling you which part connects to another? Or do you draw your own diagram?

The three main learning methods are visual, auditory, and kinesthetic. Determining which type of learner you are will help you create tools for studying.

Visual learners need to *see* the information in the form of maps, pictures, text, or math problems. Outlining notes and important points in colorful highlighters and taking note of diagrams and pictures may be key in helping you study.

Auditory learners retain information when they can *hear* directions, the spelling of a word, a math theorem, or poem. Repeating information aloud or listening to your notes on a tape recorder may help. Many auditory learners also find working in study groups or having someone quiz them is beneficial.

Kinesthetic learners must *do*! They might need to draw diagrams, write directions, or build a model. Rewriting notes on index cards or making margin notes in your textbooks also helps kinesthetic learners to retain information.

Mnemonics

Mnemonics are memory tricks that help you remember what you need to know. The three basic principles in the use of mnemonics are imagination, association, and location. Acronyms (words created from the first letters in a series of words) are common mnemonics. One acronym you may already know is **HOMES**, for the names of the Great Lakes (**H**uron, **O**ntario, **M**ichigan, **E**rie, and **S**uperior). **ROY G. BIV** reminds people of the colors in the spectrum (**R**ed, **O**range, **Y**ellow, **G**reen, **B**lue, **I**ndigo, and **V**iolet). Depending on the type of learner you are, mnemonics can also be colorful or vivid images, stories, word associations, or catchy rhymes such as "Thirty days hath September . . ." created in your mind. Any type of learner, whether visual, auditory, or kinesthetic, can use mnemonics to help the brain store and interpret information.

Step 5: Learn to Manage Your Time

Activities: Practice these strategies as you take the sample tests in this book.
Steps 5, 6, and 7 of the LearningExpress Test Preparation System put you in charge of your exam by showing you test-taking strategies that work. Practice these strategies as you take the sample tests in this book, and then you will be ready to use them on test day.

First, you will take control of your time on the exam. Most nursing assistant exams have a time limit, which may give you more than enough time to complete all the questions—or may not. It is a terrible feeling to hear the examiner say, "Five minutes left," when you are only three-quarters of the way through the test. Here are some tips to keep that from happening to you.

- **Follow directions.** If the directions are given orally, listen to them. If they are written on the exam booklet, read them carefully. Ask questions before the exam begins if there's anything you don't understand. If you are allowed to write in your exam booklet, write down the beginning time and the ending time of the exam.
- **Pace yourself.** Glance at your watch every few minutes, and compare the time to how far you have gotten in the test. When one-quarter of the time has elapsed, you should be a quarter of the way through the test, and so on. If you are falling behind, pick up the pace a bit.
- **Keep moving.** Don't spend too much time on one question. If you don't know the answer, skip the question and move on. Circle the number of the question in your test booklet in case you have time to come back to it later.
- **Keep track of your place on the answer sheet.** If you skip a question, make sure that you also skip the question on the answer sheet. Check yourself every 5–10 questions to make sure that the number of the question still corresponds with the number on the answer sheet.
- **Don't rush.** Though you should keep moving, rushing won't help. Try to keep calm and work methodically and quickly.

Step 6: Learn to Use the Process of Elimination

Activity: Complete worksheet on Using the Process of Elimination (see page 22).
After time management, your next most important tool for taking control of your exam is using the process of elimination wisely. It is standard test-taking wisdom that you should always read all the answer choices before choosing your answer. This helps you find the right answer by eliminating wrong answer choices. And, sure enough, that standard wisdom applies to your nursing assistant exam, too.

Let's say you are facing a question that goes like this:

Which of the following lists of signs and symptoms indicates a possible heart attack?
a. headache, dizziness, nausea, confusion
b. dull chest pain, sudden sweating, difficulty breathing
c. wheezing, labored breathing, chest pain
d. difficulty breathing, high fever, rapid pulse

You should always use the process of elimination on a question like this, even if the right answer jumps out at you. Sometimes the answer that jumps out isn't right after all. Let's assume, for the purpose of this exercise, that you are a little rusty on your signs and symptoms of a heart attack, so you need to use a little intuition to make up for what you don't remember. Proceed through the answer choices in order.

- **Start with choice a.** This one is pretty easy to eliminate; none of these signs and symptoms is likely to indicate a heart attack. Mark an **X** next to choice **a** so you never have to look at it again.
- **On to choice b.** "Dull chest pain" looks good, though if you are not up on your cardiac signs and symptoms, you might wonder if it should be "acute chest pain" instead. "Sudden sweating" and "difficulty breathing"? Check. And that's what you write next to choice **b**—a check mark, meaning "good answer, I might use this one."
- **Choice c is a possibility.** Maybe you don't really expect wheezing in a heart attack victim, but you know "chest pain" is right, and let's say you are not sure whether "labored breathing" is a sign of cardiac difficulty. Put a question mark next to **c**, meaning "well, maybe."
- **Choice d is also a possibility.** "Difficulty breathing" is a good sign of a heart attack. But wait a minute. "High fever?" Not really. "Rapid pulse?" Well, maybe. This doesn't really sound like a heart attack, and you have already got a better answer

picked out in choice **b**. If you are feeling sure of yourself, put an **X** next to this one. If you want to be careful, put a question mark. Now your question looks like this:

Which of the following lists of signs and symptoms indicates a possible heart attack?
X a. headache, dizziness, nausea, confusion
✓ b. dull chest pain, sudden sweating, difficulty breathing
? c. wheezing, labored breathing, chest pain
? d. difficulty breathing, high fever, rapid pulse

You have just one check mark, for a good answer. If you are pressed for time, you should simply mark choice **b** on your answer sheet. If you have the time to be extra careful, you could compare your check mark answer to your question-mark answers to make sure that it is better.

It is good to have a system for marking good, bad, and maybe answers. We recommend this one:

X = bad
✓ = good
? = maybe

If you don't like these marks, devise your own system. Just make sure you do it long before test day—while you are working through the practice exams in this book—so you are comfortable using it during the test.

Key Words

Often, identifying key words in a question will help you in the process of elimination. Words such as *always, never, all, only, must,* and *will* often make statements incorrect. Here is an example of an incorrect statement:

When a nursing assistant is preparing to ambulate a client, making sure the client is wearing proper footwear will always prevent them from falling.

The word *always* in this statement makes it incorrect. Nursing assistants must also take other measures, in addition to providing proper footwear, when ambulating a resident, such as proper body mechanics and providing support to the client.

Words like *usually, may, sometimes,* and *most* may make a statement correct. Here is an example of a correct statement:

Clients of healthcare facilities and hospitals may need help with tasks such as being fed and bathed.

The word *may* makes this statement correct. There are clients in facilities who may be too ill or weak to perform daily tasks such as feeding and bathing themselves.

Even when you think you are absolutely clueless about a question, you can often use the process of elimination to get rid of at least one answer choice. If so, you are better prepared to make an educated guess, as you will see in Step 7. More often, you can eliminate choices until you have only two possible answers. Then you are in a strong position to guess.

Try using your powers of elimination on the questions in the worksheet on the following page, Using the Process of Elimination. The questions are not about healthcare work; they are just designed to show you how the process of elimination works. The answer explanations for this worksheet show one possible way you might use the process to arrive at the right answer.

Step 7: Know When to Guess

Activity: Complete worksheet on Your Guessing Ability (see page 23).
Armed with the process of elimination, you are ready to take control of one of the big questions in test taking: Should I guess? The answer is *Yes*. Some exams have what's called a "guessing penalty," in which a fraction of your wrong answers is subtracted from your right answers—but nursing assistant exams don't tend to work like that. The number of questions you answer correctly yields your raw score. So you have nothing to lose and everything to gain by guessing.

The more complicated answer to the question "Should I guess?" depends on you—your personality and your "guessing intuition." There are two things you need to know about yourself before you go into the exam:

1. Are you a risk-taker?
2. Are you a good guesser?

You will have to decide about your risk-taking quotient on your own. To find out if you are a good guesser, complete the Your Guessing Ability worksheet on page 23.

Step 8: Reach Your Peak Performance Zone

Activity: Complete the Physical Preparation Checklist.
To get ready for a challenge like a big exam, you have to take control of your physical, as well as your mental, state. Exercise, proper diet, and rest in the weeks prior to the test will ensure that your body works with, rather than against, your mind on test day and during your preparation.

Exercise
If you don't already have a regular exercise program going, the time during which you are preparing for an exam is actually an excellent time to start one. And if you are already keeping fit—or trying to get that way—don't let the pressure of preparing for an exam fool you into quitting now. Exercise helps reduce stress by pumping feel-good hormones called endorphins into your system. It also increases the oxygen supply throughout your body, including your brain, so you will be at peak performance on test day.

A half hour of vigorous activity—enough to raise a sweat—every day should be your aim. If you are really pressed for time, every other day is okay. Choose an activity you like and get out there and do it.

USING THE PROCESS OF ELIMINATION

Use the process of elimination to answer the following questions.

1. Ilsa is as old as Meghan will be in five years. The difference between Ed's age and Meghan's age is twice the difference between Ilsa's age and Meghan's age. Ed is 29. How old is Ilsa?
   a. 4
   b. 10
   c. 19
   d. 24

2. "All drivers of commercial vehicles must carry a valid commercial driver's license whenever operating a commercial vehicle."

   According to this sentence, which of the following people need NOT carry a commercial driver's license?
   a. a truck driver idling his engine while waiting to be directed to a loading dock
   b. a bus operator backing her bus out of the way of another bus in the bus lot
   c. a taxi driver driving his personal car to the grocery store
   d. a limousine driver taking the limousine to her home after dropping off her last passenger of the evening

3. Smoking tobacco has been linked to
   a. increased risk of stroke and heart attack.
   b. all forms of respiratory disease.
   c. increasing mortality rates over the past ten years.
   d. juvenile delinquency.

4. Which of the following words is spelled correctly?
   a. incorrigible
   b. outragous
   c. domestickated
   d. understandible

Answers

Here are the answers, as well as some suggestions as to how you might have used the process of elimination to find them.

1. **d.** You should have eliminated choice **a** right off the bat. Ilsa can't be four years old if Meghan is going to be Ilsa's age in five years. The best way to eliminate other answer choices is to try plugging them in to the information given in the problem. For instance, for choice **b**, if Ilsa is 10, then Meghan must be 5. The difference between their ages is 5. The difference between Ed's age, 29, and Meghan's age, 5, is 24. Is 24 two times 5? No. Then choice **b** is wrong. You could eliminate choice **c** in the same way and be left with choice **d**.

2. **c.** Note the word *not* in the question, and go through the answers one by one. Is the truck driver in choice **a** "operating a commercial vehicle"? Yes, idling counts as "operating," so he needs to have a commercial driver's license. Likewise, the bus operator in choice **b** is operating a commercial vehicle; the question doesn't say the operator has to be on the street. The limo driver in choice **d** is operating

a commercial vehicle, even if it doesn't have a passenger in it. However, the driver in choice **c** is not operating a commercial vehicle, but his own private car.

3. a. You could eliminate choice **b** simply because of the presence of the word *all*. Such absolutes hardly ever appear in correct answer choices. Choice **c** looks attractive until you think a little about what you know—aren't fewer people smoking these days, rather than more? So how could smoking be responsible for a higher mortality rate? (If you didn't know that mortality rate means the rate at which people die, you might keep this choice as a possibility, but you would still be able to eliminate two answers and have only two to choose from.) And choice **d** is plain silly, so you could eliminate that one, too. You are left with the correct choice, **a**.

4. a. How you used the process of elimination here depends on which words you recognized as being spelled incorrectly. If you knew that the correct spellings were *outrageous*, *domesticated*, and *understandable*, then you were home free.

YOUR GUESSING ABILITY

The following are ten really hard questions. You are not supposed to know the answers. Rather, this is an assessment of your ability to guess when you don't have a clue. Read each question carefully, as if you were expected to answer it. If you have any knowledge of the subject, use that knowledge to help you eliminate wrong answer choices.

1. September 7 is Independence Day in
  a. India.
  b. Costa Rica.
  c. Brazil.
  d. Australia.

2. Which of the following is the formula for determining the momentum of an object?
  a. $p = MV$
  b. $F = ma$
  c. $P = IV$
  d. $E = mc^2$

3. Because of the expansion of the universe, the stars and other celestial bodies are all moving away from each other. This phenomenon is known as
  a. Newton's first law.
  b. the big bang.
  c. gravitational collapse.
  d. Hubble flow.

4. American author Gertrude Stein was born in
  a. 1713.
  b. 1830.
  c. 1874.
  d. 1901.

5. Which of the following is NOT one of the Five Classics attributed to Confucius?
  a. *I Ching*
  b. *Book of Holiness*
  c. *Spring and Autumn Annals*
  d. *Book of History*

6. The religious and philosophical doctrine that holds that the universe is constantly in a struggle between good and evil is known as
  a. Pelagianism.
  b. Manichaeanism.
  c. neo-Hegelianism.
  d. Epicureanism.

7. The third Chief Justice of the U.S. Supreme Court was
  a. John Blair.
  b. William Cushing.
  c. James Wilson.
  d. John Jay.

8. Which of the following is the poisonous portion of a daffodil?
  a. the bulb
  b. the leaves
  c. the stem
  d. the flowers

9. The winner of the Masters golf tournament in 1953 was
  a. Sam Snead.
  b. Cary Middlecoff.
  c. Arnold Palmer.
  d. Ben Hogan.

10. The state with the highest per capita personal income in 1980 was
  a. Alaska.
  b. Connecticut.
  c. New York.
  d. Texas.

Answers
Check your answers against the following correct answers.
  1. c.
  2. a.
  3. d.
  4. c.
  5. b.
  6. b.
  7. b.
  8. a.
  9. d.
  10. a.

How Did You Do?
You may have simply gotten lucky and actually known the answer to one or two questions. In addition, your guessing was probably more successful if you were able to use the process of elimination on any of the questions. Maybe you didn't know who the third Chief Justice was (question 7), but you knew that John Jay was the first. In that case, you would have eliminated choice **d** and, therefore, improved your odds of guessing right from one in four to one in three.

According to probability, you should get two-and-a-half answers correct, so getting either two or three right would be average. If you got four or more right, you may be a really terrific guesser. If you got one or none right, you may be a really bad guesser.

Keep in mind, though, that this is only a small sample. You should continue to keep track of your guessing ability as you work through the sample questions in this book. Circle the numbers of questions you guess on as you make your guess; or, if you don't have time while you take the practice tests, go back afterward and try to remember which questions you guessed at. Remember, on a test with four answer choices, your chance of guessing correctly is one in four. So keep a separate "guessing" score for each exam. How many questions did you guess on? How many did you get right? If the number you got right is at least one-fourth of the number of questions you guessed on, you are at least an average guesser—maybe better—and you should always go ahead and guess on the real exam. If the number you got right is significantly lower than one-fourth of the number you guessed on, you would be safe in guessing anyway, but maybe you would feel more comfortable if you guessed only selectively, when you can eliminate a wrong answer or at least have a good feeling about one of the answer choices.

Remember, even if you are a play-it-safe person with lousy intuition, you are still safe guessing every time.

Jogging with a friend always makes the time go faster, or take a portable music player.

But don't overdo it. You don't want to exhaust yourself. Moderation is the key.

Diet

First of all, cut out the junk. Go easy on caffeine and nicotine, and eliminate alcohol from your system at least two weeks before the exam. What your body needs for peak performance is simply a balanced diet. Eat plenty of fruits and vegetables, along with protein and carbohydrates.

Make sure to eat a healthy breakfast the day of the exam. Be sure to include protein, complex carbohydrates, and some fat. Complex carbohydrates, such as whole-grain toast or oatmeal, help you feel energized throughout the day.

Rest

You probably know how much sleep you need every night to be at your best, even if you don't always get it. Make sure you do get that much sleep, though, for at least a week before the exam. Moderation is important here, too. Extra sleep will just make you groggy.

If you are not a morning person and your exam will be given in the morning, you should reset your internal clock so that your body doesn't think you are taking an exam at 3 a.m. You have to start this process well before the exam. The way it works is to get up half an hour earlier each morning, and then go to bed half an hour earlier that night. Don't try it the other way around; you will just toss and turn if you go to bed early without having gotten up early. The next morning, get up another half an hour earlier, and so on. How long you will have to do this depends on how late you are used to getting up.

Step 9: Get Your Act Together

Activity: Complete the Final Preparations worksheet. You are in control of your mind and body; you are in charge of test anxiety, your preparation, and your test-taking strategies. Now it is time to take charge of external factors, like the testing site and the materials you need to take the exam.

Find Out Where the Test Is and Make a Trial Run

The testing agency or your nursing assistant instructor will notify you when and where your exam is being held. Do you know how to get to the testing site? Do you know how long it will take to get there? If not, make a trial run, preferably on the same day of the week at the same time of day. Make note, on the Final Preparations worksheet on page 27, of the amount of time it will take you to get to the exam site. Plan on arriving at least 10–15 minutes early so you can get the lay of the land, use the bathroom, and calm down. Then figure out how early you will have to get up that morning, and make sure you get up that early every day for a week before the exam.

Gather Your Materials

The night before the exam, lay out the clothes you will wear and the materials you have to bring with you to the exam. Plan on dressing in layers; you won't have any control over the temperature of the examination room. Have a sweater or jacket you can take off if it is warm. Use the checklist on the Final Preparations worksheet on page 27 to help you pull together what you will need.

Don't Skip Breakfast

Even if you don't usually eat breakfast, do so on exam morning. A cup of coffee doesn't count. Don't eat doughnuts or other sweet foods, either. A sugar high will leave you with a sugar low in the middle of the exam. A mix of protein and complex carbohydrates is best: Cereal with milk, or eggs with whole-grain toast, will do your body a world of good.

Step 10: Do It!

Activity: Ace the nursing assistant exam!

Fast forward to exam day. You are ready. You made a study plan and followed through. You practiced your test-taking strategies while working through this book. You are in control of your physical, mental, and emotional states. You know when and where to show up and what to bring with you. In other words, you are better prepared than most of the other people taking the nursing assistant exam with you. You are psyched.

Just one more thing. . . . When you are done with the exam, you deserve a reward. Plan a celebration. Call up your friends and plan a party, or have a nice dinner for two—whatever your heart desires. Give yourself something to look forward to.

And then do it. Go into the exam, full of confidence, armed with test-taking strategies you have practiced until they are second nature. You are in control of yourself, your environment, and your performance on the exam. You are ready to succeed. So do it. Go in there and ace the exam. And look forward to your future career as a nursing assistant!

Getting to the Exam Site

Location of exam site: _____

Date: _____

Departure time: _____

Do I know how to get to the exam site?   Yes ___   No ___   (If no, make a trial run.)

Time it will take to get to exam site _____

Things to Lay Out the Night Before

Clothes I will wear   ___

Sweater/jacket   ___

Watch   ___

Photo ID   ___

Four #2 pencils   ___

Other Things to Bring/Remember

_____   _____

_____   _____

_____   _____

_____   _____

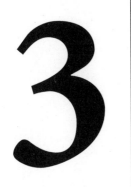

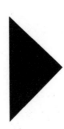

NURSING ASSISTANT/NURSE AIDE PRACTICE EXAM 1

CHAPTER SUMMARY

This is the first of five practice exams in this book based on the National Nurse Aide Assessment Program (NNAAP) written exam. Use this first test to identify your areas of strength and weakness.

f you are required to take a written exam in order to be certified, the exam you take is likely to be very much like this one, based on the NNAAP. This exam has 70 multiple-choice questions covering the range of duties performed by a certified nursing assistant:

- **Physical Care Skills**—activities of daily living, basic nursing skills, restorative skills
- **Psychosocial Care Skills**—emotional- and mental-health needs, spiritual and cultural needs
- **Role of the Nurse Aide**—communication, client rights, legal and ethical behavior as a member of the healthcare team

As with the NNAAP, this exam is not divided into these sections; you may find questions on very different topics right next to each other.

Normally you would have two hours to complete a test like this, but for now, don't worry about timing. Just answer all of the questions in one sitting. The answer sheet you should use for filling in your answers is on the next page. After the exam is an answer key, with all the answers explained. These explanations will help you see your areas of strength and weakness. Then you will know which parts of your training materials to study before you take the second practice exam. You can refer to the Appendix (page 159) for a breakdown of the question types. The chart will help you understand which kinds of questions are most difficult for you, so you can focus on those skills for next time. Generally, a score of 75% or higher is considered passing.

Practice Exam 1

1.	(a)	(b)	(c)	(d)
2.	(a)	(b)	(c)	(d)
3.	(a)	(b)	(c)	(d)
4.	(a)	(b)	(c)	(d)
5.	(a)	(b)	(c)	(d)
6.	(a)	(b)	(c)	(d)
7.	(a)	(b)	(c)	(d)
8.	(a)	(b)	(c)	(d)
9.	(a)	(b)	(c)	(d)
10.	(a)	(b)	(c)	(d)
11.	(a)	(b)	(c)	(d)
12.	(a)	(b)	(c)	(d)
13.	(a)	(b)	(c)	(d)
14.	(a)	(b)	(c)	(d)
15.	(a)	(b)	(c)	(d)
16.	(a)	(b)	(c)	(d)
17.	(a)	(b)	(c)	(d)
18.	(a)	(b)	(c)	(d)
19.	(a)	(b)	(c)	(d)
20.	(a)	(b)	(c)	(d)
21.	(a)	(b)	(c)	(d)
22.	(a)	(b)	(c)	(d)
23.	(a)	(b)	(c)	(d)
24.	(a)	(b)	(c)	(d)
25.	(a)	(b)	(c)	(d)

26.	(a)	(b)	(c)	(d)
27.	(a)	(b)	(c)	(d)
28.	(a)	(b)	(c)	(d)
29.	(a)	(b)	(c)	(d)
30.	(a)	(b)	(c)	(d)
31.	(a)	(b)	(c)	(d)
32.	(a)	(b)	(c)	(d)
33.	(a)	(b)	(c)	(d)
34.	(a)	(b)	(c)	(d)
35.	(a)	(b)	(c)	(d)
36.	(a)	(b)	(c)	(d)
37.	(a)	(b)	(c)	(d)
38.	(a)	(b)	(c)	(d)
39.	(a)	(b)	(c)	(d)
40.	(a)	(b)	(c)	(d)
41.	(a)	(b)	(c)	(d)
42.	(a)	(b)	(c)	(d)
43.	(a)	(b)	(c)	(d)
44.	(a)	(b)	(c)	(d)
45.	(a)	(b)	(c)	(d)
46.	(a)	(b)	(c)	(d)
47.	(a)	(b)	(c)	(d)
48.	(a)	(b)	(c)	(d)
49.	(a)	(b)	(c)	(d)
50.	(a)	(b)	(c)	(d)

51.	(a)	(b)	(c)	(d)
52.	(a)	(b)	(c)	(d)
53.	(a)	(b)	(c)	(d)
54.	(a)	(b)	(c)	(d)
55.	(a)	(b)	(c)	(d)
56.	(a)	(b)	(c)	(d)
57.	(a)	(b)	(c)	(d)
58.	(a)	(b)	(c)	(d)
59.	(a)	(b)	(c)	(d)
60.	(a)	(b)	(c)	(d)
61.	(a)	(b)	(c)	(d)
62.	(a)	(b)	(c)	(d)
63.	(a)	(b)	(c)	(d)
64.	(a)	(b)	(c)	(d)
65.	(a)	(b)	(c)	(d)
66.	(a)	(b)	(c)	(d)
67.	(a)	(b)	(c)	(d)
68.	(a)	(b)	(c)	(d)
69.	(a)	(b)	(c)	(d)
70.	(a)	(b)	(c)	(d)

Practice Exam 1

1. When assisting a client in learning how to use a cane, the nurse aide stands
   a. approximately two feet directly behind the client.
   b. about one foot from the client's weak side.
   c. about one foot from the client's strong side.
   d. slightly behind the client on the client's weak side.

2. When working with a client who has urinary retention, the nurse aide can expect that the client will
   a. urinate large volumes.
   b. be unable to urinate.
   c. urinate frequently.
   d. be incontinent of urine.

3. Aging-related hearing changes result in older clients gradually losing their ability to hear
   a. high-pitched sounds.
   b. low-pitched sounds.
   c. sound levels.
   d. faint sounds.

4. The best way to safely identify your patient is by
   a. asking his name.
   b. calling his name and waiting for his response.
   c. checking the bed plate.
   d. checking the name tag.

5. A client is on a bowel and bladder training program and has not had a bowel movement in three days. The nurse aide should
   a. report it to the charge nurse.
   b. give the client an enema.
   c. offer the client prune juice.
   d. encourage the client to drink more fluids.

6. The proper medical abbreviation for before meals is
   a. p.c.
   b. b.i.d.
   c. a.c.
   d. t.i.d.

7. A client diagnosed with hypertension will most likely have a history of
   a. low blood pressure.
   b. high blood pressure.
   c. low blood sugar.
   d. high blood sugar.

8. A patient who has difficulty chewing or swallowing will need what type of diet?
   a. clear liquid
   b. low residue
   c. pureed
   d. mechanical soft

9. An elderly resident with Alzheimer's disease cannot find her room. How can the nurse aide help the client feel more independent?
   a. Tell her to stay in the room.
   b. Have her roommate secretly watch her.
   c. Place a familiar object on the client's door.
   d. Write the room number on a piece of paper.

10. How often should a patient's intake and output records be totaled?
   a. once each shift
   b. twice a day
   c. every four hours
   d. every 12 hours

11. Which of the following should the nursing assistant observe and record when admitting a client?

   a. freckles

   b. wrinkles

   c. short nails

   d. bruises

12. When responding to a client on the intercom, the nursing assistant should say

   a. "Hello, who is calling, please?"

   b. "What is it that you want?"

   c. "This is [nursing assistant name and position], can I help you?"

   d. "Please hold; I'll have the nurse answer your call."

13. Which of the following things should the nurse aide do to familiarize new clients with their surroundings?

   a. Demonstrate the location and use of the call light.

   b. Explain that the TV is not to be used.

   c. Instruct family to leave the room after the aide is finished with the admission.

   d. Raise the bed to the high position and raise the safety rails.

14. When arranging a client's room, the nursing assistant should do all of the following EXCEPT

   a. checking the placement of the call bell.

   b. adjusting the back rest as directed.

   c. administering the client's medications.

   d. adjusting the lighting as appropriate.

15. When assisting a client out of bed, the nurse aide should always

   a. employ body mechanic techniques.

   b. get another nurse aide to assist.

   c. raise the bed to its maximum height.

   d. lower all safety rails.

16. How often should clients be repositioned during an eight-hour shift?

   a. q1h

   b. q2h

   c. q3h

   d. q4h

17. Which of the following is the correct procedure for serving a meal to a client who must be fed?

   a. Serve the tray along with all the other trays, and then come back to feed the client.

   b. Bring the tray to the client first, and feed the client before serving the other clients.

   c. Bring the tray into the room when you are ready to feed the client.

   d. Have the kitchen hold the tray for one hour.

18. The most serious problem that wrinkles in the bedclothes can cause is

   a. restlessness.

   b. sleeplessness.

   c. decubitus ulcers.

   d. bleeding and shock.

19. Restorative care begins

   a. as soon as possible.

   b. when the client is ready.

   c. when the client is discharged.

   d. when the client is diagnosed as terminally ill.

20. Before placing a client in Fowler's position, the nurse aide should

   a. turn the client onto her abdomen.

   b. explain the procedure to the client.

   c. flatten the entire bed.

   d. remake the bed with new linens.

21. During handwashing, the nurse aiden accidentally touches the inside of the sink while rinsing the soap off. The next action is to
   a. allow the water to run over the hands for two minutes.
   b. dry the hands and turn off the faucet with the paper towel.
   c. repeat the wash from the beginning.
   d. repeat washing, but for half the time.

22. How should a nurse aide dress for a job interview?
   a. wearing a clean t-shirt and casual slacks
   b. wearing a nurse aide uniform
   c. wearing a business suit, dress, or pants and dress shirt
   d. wearing formal attire

23. An ambulatory client is newly admitted. Before leaving the client alone, the nurse aide should
   a. ask if the client is hungry.
   b. inspect the client's skin.
   c. assess the client's intake and output.
   d. make sure the client knows how to use the call bell.

24. When lifting a heavy object, the correct method would be to bend at the
   a. waist, keeping your legs straight.
   b. waist, rounding your shoulders.
   c. knees, keeping your back straight.
   d. knees and waist.

25. When should nurse aides wash their hands?
   a. before eating
   b. before using the bathroom
   c. after client care
   d. before cleaning a bedpan

26. When assisting a client with eating, one of the first things the nurse aide should do is
   a. cut the food into bite-size pieces.
   b. wash his own hands and the client's hands.
   c. butter the client's bread.
   d. provide the client with privacy.

27. A patient has a new cast on her right arm. While caring for her, it is important to first observe for
   a. pulse above the cast.
   b. color and hardness of the cast.
   c. warmth and color of fingers.
   d. signs of crumbling at the cast end.

28. Encouraging a client to take part in activities of daily living (ADLs) such as bathing, combing hair, and feeding is
   a. done only when time permits.
   b. the family's responsibility.
   c. necessary for rehabilitation.
   d. a violation of client rights.

29. In caring for a confused elderly man, it is important to remember to
   a. keep the bedrails up except when you are at the bedside.
   b. close the door to the room so that he does not disturb other patients.
   c. keep the room dark and quiet at all times to keep the patient from becoming upset.
   d. remind him each morning to shower and shave independently.

30. Before assisting a client into a wheelchair, the first action would be to check if the
   a. client is adequately covered.
   b. floor is slippery.
   c. door to the room is closed.
   d. wheels of the chair are locked.

31. A client has a weak left side. When transferring the client from the bed to the wheelchair, the nurse aide should stand
a. on the right side.
b. in front of the client.
c. on the left side.
d. behind the client.

32. While making rounds at 5:30 a.m., a nurse aide finds a patient lying on the floor. What should the nurse aide do first?
a. Call 911.
b. Perform CPR.
c. Call for help.
d. Assess the client's pulse and respirations.

33. When moving a wheelchair onto an elevator, the nurse aide should stay
a. behind the chair and pull it toward the aide.
b. behind the chair and push it away from the aide.
c. in front of the client to observe the client's condition.
d. at the side of the wheelchair while opening the door.

34. The Foley bag must be kept lower than the client's bladder so that
a. urine will not leak out, soiling the bed.
b. urine will not return to the bladder, causing infection.
c. the bag will be hidden and the client will not be embarrassed.
d. the client will be more comfortable in bed.

35. As an afternoon snack, the kitchen sent a diabetic client a container of chocolate ice cream. The nursing assistant should first
a. substitute diet soda for the ice cream.
b. hold the afternoon snack and report to the charge nurse.
c. call the kitchen and report the error.
d. allow the client to have half of the ice cream.

36. When assisting a client who is using the commode, it is important to
a. leave the call light within reach.
b. lock the door to promote privacy.
c. stand next to the client until the client is finished.
d. restrain the client to prevent a fall.

37. Ensuring adequate circulation to tissues is a major factor in preventing skin breakdown. This can be accomplished by doing all of the following EXCEPT
a. positioning the patient every four hours.
b. using mechanical aids.
c. giving backrubs.
d. performing active or passive ROM exercises.

38. The purpose of cold applications is usually to
a. speed the flow of blood to the area.
b. prevent heat exhaustion.
c. prevent or reduce swelling.
d. prevent the formation of scar tissue.

39. The hot water bottle is an example of a
a. local dry heat application.
b. generalized dry heat application.
c. local moist heat application.
d. generalized moist heat application.

40. Clients receiving an enema are usually placed
    a. on the right side.
    b. on the left side.
    c. flat on the back.
    d. in a semisitting position.

41. A female client's perineal area should be cleansed before which specimen is collected?
    a. 24-hour urine specimen
    b. midstream clean-catch urine specimen
    c. pediatric routine urine specimen
    d. routine urine specimen

42. The most common site for counting the pulse is the
    a. carotid artery.
    b. femoral artery.
    c. brachial artery.
    d. radial artery.

43. When counting respirations, the nurse aide should
    a. wait until after the client has exercised.
    b. not tell the patient what he is going to do.
    c. count five respirations and then check his watch.
    d. have the client count respirations while the aide takes her pulse.

44. Which of the following is NOT the nurse aide's responsibility when caring for clients who have urinary catheters?
    a. inserting the catheter
    b. ensuring that the catheter drains properly
    c. preventing infection
    d. recording urinary output

45. When giving information to the charge nurse for an incident report, the nurse aide should
    a. write in the client's chart that an incident occurred.
    b. keep the report in her personal file.
    c. state the facts clearly.
    d. give her opinions as to the cause of the incident.

46. All long-term care nurse aides must be competency evaluated and must complete a distinct educational course. These requirements are set by
    a. OBRA '87.
    b. OSHA.
    c. CDC.
    d. FDA.

47. A resident is blind. It is important not to
    a. leave the door completely closed.
    b. rearrange the furniture.
    c. announce yourself before entering the room.
    d. explain the location of food on the plate, using the face of the clock to assist.

48. When family members visit a client, the visitors should
    a. stay in the day room.
    b. stay a short while so as not to tire the client.
    c. be expected to help with care.
    d. be allowed privacy with the client.

49. A resident asks, "If I need help during the night, who will be there?" The nursing assistant should respond,
    a. "Don't worry, you'll be okay."
    b. "Just yell; someone will hear you."
    c. "Your roommate will probably ring the call bell."
    d. "There are people here all night to help you."

50. Which of the following is a client's right?
a. having personal information kept confidential
b. obtaining private duty staff if desired
c. knowing what is wrong with the client's roommate
d. treating the staff any way he or she pleases

51. A resident often cries while she is receiving her p.m. care. What should the nurse aide do?
a. Tell her to stop crying.
b. Ignore her and continue with her care.
c. Tell her jokes to make her laugh.
d. Tell her that it's all right to cry, and that the aide is there for her if she wants to talk.

52. When providing denture care, the nurse aide must
a. wash them in boiling water.
b. hold them under warm running water.
c. dunk them in and out of cool water.
d. place them on a towel in the sink with cool water.

53. Sexuality in long-term care clients may include all of the following EXCEPT
a. needing private time with a partner.
b. caring about one's physical appearance.
c. engaging in public fondling.
d. desiring sexual interaction.

54. A client is scheduled for a partial bed bath. This means that the nurse aide must wash the client's
a. face, neck, ears, arms, and hands.
b. face, axillae, hands, and buttocks.
c. face, hands, axillae, and legs.
d. face, hands, axillae, genitals, and buttocks.

55. A goal for an extended care facility (ECF) resident is that she not swear at the nurses or aides. When she calls an aide by his name, the appropriate action is to
a. smile and give the appropriate reward.
b. continue whatever task that is being done.
c. tease the resident about not swearing.
d. tell all of the staff that she didn't swear.

56. An agitated resident must be turned every two hours all night long. The first action of the nurse aide when waking up this resident is to
a. turn on the light.
b. speak quietly and calmly.
c. touch her shoulder.
d. shout her name.

57. If a client objects to certain food for religious or cultural reasons, the appropriate action would be to
a. tell him to wait for the next meal.
b. offer to substitute something different for him.
c. call the dietician the next day.
d. tell him he needs to eat what is on his tray.

58. The client's religion forbids eating pork. Bacon is being served for breakfast. The most appropriate response is to
a. encourage the client to eat it because she needs protein.
b. tell the client it is all right since her doctor ordered the diet.
c. call the kitchen for a tray without bacon.
d. tell the client that restrictions are not as important as her health.

59. Which type of communication can often be most powerful?
  a. written
  b. verbal
  c. silent
  d. tactile

60. A client refuses to allow the nurse aide to bathe her. The nurse aide tells the client that she will not be allowed to eat lunch or go to bingo if she does not have her bath. This is an example of
  a. rehabilitation.
  b. discipline.
  c. verbal abuse.
  d. physical abuse.

61. On entering a room, an aide notices that the client is not breathing. The aide's first action should be to
  a. call for help.
  b. lay the client down on his back.
  c. give four quick breaths.
  d. give 8–10 abdominal thrusts.

62. A client's dentures are lost. The first action should be to
  a. notify the administrator.
  b. look for them.
  c. notify the doctor.
  d. notify the charge nurse.

63. Nursing assistants are responsible for
  a. planning client care.
  b. doing tasks assigned by the charge nurse.
  c. performing without ever asking for help.
  d. comparing assignments with coworkers.

64. A patient turns on the call light when he needs to urinate. The appropriate action is to
  a. ignore the light, since he is not the aide's own client.
  b. announce on the intercom that there are two patients ahead of him.
  c. answer the call light and get the urinal.
  d. answer the call light when the aide has the time.

65. A client is on CMR and in the prone position. The nurse aide finds the client vomiting bright red blood. The nurse aide should first
  a. clean up the vomit.
  b. place the client in the side-lying position.
  c. provide the client with an emesis basin.
  d. call the charge nurse.

66. When performing catheter care, the nurse aide should wash the catheter
  a. toward the meatus.
  b. with Betadine soap.
  c. away from the meatus.
  d. with alcohol.

67. A nurse aide who applies restraints on a client without directions from the charge nurse may be accused of
  a. slander.
  b. battery.
  c. false imprisonment.
  d. negligence.

68. H.S. care is care that is given
  a. before meals.
  b. before bedtime.
  c. after meals.
  d. upon awakening.

69. The best food choices for a geriatric client with no teeth would include
   a. hamburger, french fries, corn, and ice cream.
   b. baked chicken, dressing, green beans, and coconut macaroons.
   c. spare ribs, macaroni and cheese, coleslaw, and fruit cocktail.
   d. baked fish, whipped potatoes, spinach soufflé, and tapioca.

70. A client's family wants to talk about the client's impending death, but the client does not want to talk about it. The family should be encouraged to
   a. carry on the conversation away from the client.
   b. talk freely in front of the client in order to help the client to accept it.
   c. wait until the client dies to talk about it.
   d. force the client to talk about it with them.

Answers

1. d. Standing slightly behind the client at her weak side better enables the nurse aide to prevent falls. Choices **a** and **b** are incorrect because these distances are too far to safely catch the client if she falls or to support her. Choice **c** is incorrect because if a nurse aide is placed there, the client may collapse on her weak side.

2. b. Urinary retention means that the client cannot urinate. The problem should be reported to the nurse as soon as possible. Choice **a** is incorrect; urinating in large volumes, also called *polyuria*, is indicative of a medical problem such as diabetes mellitus. Choice **c** is incorrect; urinating too frequently means that the client may have a problem such as a urinary tract infection. Choice **d** is incorrect; urinary incontinence is the accidental release of urine. It may happen in small amounts when someone coughs or sneezes, or regularly if someone has a medical problem. While choices **a**, **c**, and **d** are not the correct answers, these problems should be reported to the nurse as soon as possible.

3. a. Age-related hearing loss, also called *presbycusis*, results in older persons gradually losing their ability to hear high-pitched sounds. Choice **b** is incorrect; the inability to hear low-pitched sounds may mean that the client has *otosclerosis*, which is usually related to abnormal bone growth in the bones of the inner ear. Choices **c** and **d** are incorrect; a reduction in sound level and the inability to hear faint sounds can indicate hearing loss due to problems such as an ear infection or impacted cerumen (too much ear wax).

4. d. Checking a client's name tag is the safest way of assuring that you have the correct client. If you ask a client his name, and he is confused or has difficulty hearing, he may give you the wrong name or not reply when you call his name. A confused client may also be lying in the wrong bed.

5. a. The nurse aide should report this problem because nurse aides cannot perform any of the interventions on their own. Nurse aides cannot give clients enemas without being instructed to do so by the nurse. They also cannot encourage drinking more fluids or give prune juice as a treatment on their own (and prune juice would be insufficient for this client).

6. c. The proper medical abbreviation for before meals is a.c., p.c. is the proper medical abbreviation for after meals, b.i.d. is the proper medical abbreviation for twice a day, and t.i.d. is the proper medical abbreviation for three times a day.

7. b. *Hypertension* is the medical term for high blood pressure, so the client will most likely have this problem in his history, although it may now be controlled with medication. The medical term for low blood pressure is *hypotension*. The medical term for low blood sugar is *hypoglycemia*. The medical term for high blood sugar is *hyperglycemia*.

8. d. A mechanical soft diet is prescribed for clients who need a diet that is easy to chew, swallow, and digest. Choice **a** is incorrect; a clear liquid diet is usually prescribed for clients before medical tests, for clients who have nausea and vomiting or an acute illness, or for clients who have just experienced trauma or surgery. Choice **b** is incorrect; a low residue diet is prescribed for clients to reduce the frequency and volume of their stools. Choice **c** is incorrect; a pureed diet is prescribed for clients who have poor dentition, who are very frail, or who are in end-stage disease.

9. c. A familiar object can enable a client to find her room on her own, helping her feel more independent. Telling a client to stay in her room is restrictive and may be a violation of her rights. Choice **b** is incorrect because asking a roommate to do something for another client is inappropriate—it puts undue strain on the roommate and can create an unsafe environment for the client and the roommate. Choice **d** is incorrect because the client may lose the piece of paper or may be too confused at times to know what the number means.

10. a. Intake and output are usually recorded every shift, as well as every 24 hours. Most agencies run on 8-hour shifts, not 12-hour shifts. When clients need more frequent observation of intake and output, they are usually ill enough to need hourly observations and may thus be in the critical care unit.

11. d. Bruising may be due to accidents, abuse, medications, or illness, and should be recorded and reported. Freckles and wrinkles are normal skin variations and do not require recording or reporting. Short nails are not problematic; however, long nails may result in the client scratching and injuring herself.

12. c. Always give your name and position when answering the call bell, and politely ask the client what she wants. Choices **a** and **b** are incorrect; these questions may come across as the nurse aide acting in a rude manner and should be avoided. Choice **d** is incorrect because it is a nurse aide's responsibility to answer call bells promptly and appropriately.

13. a. The nurse aide should make sure that the client knows how to call for help. Unless otherwise noted, the TV is there for the client to use, and unless otherwise stated, there is no reason to ask the family to leave the room once the client is admitted. Choice **d** is incorrect, because while raising the safety rails is appropriate, raising the bed to the highest position creates a dangerous situation if the client is left alone.

14. c. Nursing assistants are not allowed to administer medications. The nursing assistant should check to make sure that the call bell is within the client's reach, adjust the back rest as directed, and adjust the room lighting for comfort and visibility.

15. a. Nurse aides should always use proper body mechanics when moving clients. The nurse aide obtains the assistance of another nurse aide only when it is required. Raising the bed to the maximum height when assisting a client out of bed increases the risk of the client's falling out of the bed and injuring herself. Raised side rails can be used by the client for balance to assist her out of the bed.

16. b. Clients should be turned every two hours to prevent decubiti. Choice **a** is incorrect; unless there is a reason, turning a client every hour is too frequent and disruptive to the client's rest. Choices **c** and **d** are incorrect; turning the client every three or four hours is not frequent enough to prevent decubiti.

17. c. An aide should not bring the tray into the room until he has time to feed the client. Choice **a** is incorrect, because the client may attempt to feed herself and may choke on the food. Choice **b** is incorrect, because it takes time to feed a client and thus the other clients will be waiting too long to receive their food. Choice **d** is incorrect, because the food will not be palatable after sitting around for an hour.

NURSING ASSISTANT/NURSE AIDE PRACTICE EXAM 1

18. c. The most serious problem that wrinkles in the bedclothes can cause is decubitus ulcers, also called decubiti. Restlessness and sleeplessness are problematic and may cause health issues, but they are not the most serious problems. Bleeding and shock are not common complications of wrinkled bed clothing.

19. a. Restorative care begins as early as possible to prevent further disability. Choice **b** is incorrect; the planning stage of restorative care can begin before the client is ready. Choice **c** is incorrect; there will not be enough time to successfully carry out restorative care if one waits until discharge. Restorative care is not used for terminal clients. End of life care may be more appropriate.

20. b. Caregivers should always explain procedures first. Turning a client on her abdomen is using the prone position. The Fowler's position requires the nurse aide to raise the head of the bed 45 to 60 degrees. Remaking the bed is unnecessary to place a client in Fowler's position.

21. c. The aide has contaminated her hands and must rewash her hands. She must completely start over. Plain water will not remove bacteria, and the full time is required to remove the contamination from the sink.

22. c. First impressions are critical, so nurse aides should wear business attire. Choice **a** is incorrect, because the nurse aide should present himself as a well-groomed professional. Choice **b** is incorrect, because wearing a uniform outside the workplace may be disallowed in some facilities because it can become contaminated. Choice **d** is incorrect, because wearing formal attire is overdressing and not businesslike.

23. d. New clients should always know how to call for help before being left alone. Choice **a** is incorrect; the client may not be allowed to have food due to upcoming testing or surgery. Choice **b** is incorrect; it is the nurse's role to inspect the client's skin at the time of admission. Choice **c** is incorrect; the client was just admitted and thus will not have an intake or output yet.

24. c. Keeping the back straight forces the body to use strong leg muscles. Bending at the waist with legs straight can cause back injury, and bending at the waist with rounded shoulders can cause back injury.

25. c. Nurse aides should wash their hands after client care to prevent cross-contamination. Nurse aides should wash their hands *after* eating, *after* using the bathroom, and *after* cleaning a bedpan.

26. b. Nurse aides must always remember to consider infection control first before anything else. Eventually, food should be cut into 1/3-size bites to prevent choking. Choice **c** is incorrect, because the nurse aide should first ask the client if he wants butter on his bread. Choice **d** is incorrect because the client may want to eat with others to socialize.

27. c. A new cast may cut off circulation, and checking the pulse below the cast helps to make sure that this has not happened. The pulse above the cast will not help detect cast tightness. A new cast will be damp and should not be touched with fingertips to prevent pitting the cast. Crumbling should not be an issue with a new cast.

28. c. Rehabilitation should always be part of the care plan, and encouraging a client to take part in ADLs is an expected role of the nurse aide. This is the nurse aide's responsibility (however, the family can assist the client if they desire to do so and there are no contraindications). Considerate and respectful care is a basic right of all clients.

29. a. A nurse aide should always make sure to follow agency policy. Closing the door causes client isolation, and keeping the room dark and quiet at all times can cause sensory deprivation, which can increase confusion. A confused client needs assistance with bathing and shaving to avoid injury.

30. d. Before assisting a patient into a wheelchair, check to see if the wheels of the chair are locked. Making sure the client is covered is important, but not the first action. The nurse should check the floor before entering a room to avoid self-injury, and the door should be open in case the call bell falls out of reach and the nurse aide needs to call for help.

31. c. Assist the client at the client's weak side to prevent falls. Choice **a** is incorrect; the nurse aide should stand at the client's weak side, not strong one. Choice **b** is incorrect; this is done for clients who do not have one-sided weakness. Choice **d** is incorrect, because the client may slide and fall.

32. d. The nurse aide should assess pulse and breathing first. The client may have fainted. The nurse aide should check pulse and respiration status before calling for help or performing CPR.

33. a. The nurse aide must stay behind the chair to control it and move it backward to prevent the wheels from falling into the door opening. The nurse aide needs to remain near the client and in control of the wheelchair.

34. b. Raising the bag above the bladder level can lead to backflow of urine and can cause bacteria to flow into the bladder. The Foley system is a closed system and should not leak, and the bag can be hidden at almost any height. Preventing backflow does avoid discomfort, but this is secondary.

35. b. The nursing assistant should report this error to the charge nurse, who in turn will contact the kitchen to obtain the correct nourishment. The nurse aide cannot substitute food for a client with diabetes, and diet cola has no calories and is thus not a substitute for a healthy afternoon snack. It is the nurse's role to call the kitchen. Choice **d** is incorrect, because ice cream contains sugar and fat, and a diabetic snack needs to be carefully calculated into their overall diet.

36. a. The client should always have access to a means to get help when needed. A locked door slows access to the client in the event of an emergency. Standing next to the client deprives the client of privacy. Restraining a client without an order or consent can be considered unlawful imprisonment.

37. a. The patient must be positioned every *two* hours to prevent skin breakdown due to poor circulation. Certain mechanical aides are created for the purpose of preventing skin breakdown; backrubs prevent skin breakdown by stimulating circulation; and range of motion exercise improves circulation and joint mobility, thus decreasing skin breakdown.

38. c. The purpose of cold applications is usually to prevent or reduce swelling. Warm applications speed the flow of blood to an area. Cold applications are not used to prevent heat exhaustion and will not prevent scar formation.

39. a. A hot water bottle applied by itself is local dry heat. A hot water bottle is too small for generalized application.

40. b. Placing the patient on the left side allows better entry into the colon. Placing a client on the right side or on the back makes entry into the colon more difficult. A semisitting position is unstable and causes the client to fall.

41. b. The clean-catch specimen requires cleaning the perineum. A 24-hour urine specimen and a routine urine specimen do not require prior cleaning, regardless of age.

42. d. The carotid artery, femoral artery, and brachial artery are not used routinely to count a client's pulse.

43. b. Telling the patient that the aide is watching her breathing will cause the patient to slightly change her breathing pattern. Choice **a** is incorrect, because exercise will temporarily increase the client's respirations. Choice **c** is incorrect because respirations are counted over 30 or 60 seconds. Choice **d** is incorrect because clients cannot count their own respirations.

44. a. Nurse aides are not responsible for catheter insertion. Nurse aides should ensure that the catheter drains properly, take proper precautions to prevent infection, and record the urinary output when a client has a catheter.

45. c. An incident report becomes a permanent part of the legal record. Make sure the facts are clear. The nurse, not the aide, documents incident reports. The incident report becomes a hospital record, not a personal record. Incident reports require facts, not opinions.

46. a. OBRA '87 stands for Omnibus Budget Reconciliation Act of 1987. OSHA stands for Occupational Safety and Health Administration. CDC stands for Centers for Disease Control and Prevention. FDA stands for the Food and Drug Administration.

47. b. Never rearrange the f[...] patient's room after t[...] This can cause falls. [...] ents who are visually [...] same respect and privacy as those who can see clearly. Choice **c** is incorrect; announcing yourself allows the client to know that you have entered the room. Choice **d** is incorrect; explaining the location of food on the plate helps the visually impaired client to be more independent by feeding himself.

48. d. The family members should expect and be allowed private time with their loved one. Visitors should be allowed to visit directly with the client, and as long as possible, wherever appropriate. Family visitation is important to the healing and well-being of the client. Family may help with care if they wish, but should not be required to do so.

49. d. To make clients feel safe, assure them that help is always there, if needed. Telling a worried client not to worry is not helpful and can be disrespectful. Telling a client to yell for help or saying that a roommate will probably ring the bell is not helpful or reassuring.

50. a. Clients have the right to confidentiality. This means that all clients have the right to confidentiality, which includes roommates. While clients are allowed to obtain private duty staff, it is not a client right. Clients do not have a right to treat the staff with disrespect.

51. d. It is normal for a person to have moments of sadness, and it is important for the patient to know that the nurse aide cares. The nurse aide should also report this to the nurse in case the crying is the result of something more serious, such as depression. It is inappropriate to tell a client to stop crying, but at the same time, the nurse aide should not ignore clients and their needs. Humor can sometimes help, but will probably not help in cases where sadness seems frequent.

2. d. Dentures are expensive. The towel prevents breakage if dropped, and the cool water prevents warping. Choice **a** is incorrect; hot water can damage dentures. Use lukewarm water. Choice **b** is incorrect because holding them under running water runs the risk of dropping and breaking them. Choice **c** is incorrect; dentures need to be carefully cleaned to remove food debris and old denture adhesive.

53. c. As long-term care providers, nursing assistants must respect the resident's right to sexuality. However, engaging in public fondling is inappropriate and may infringe on other resident's rights. Private time with a partner is appropriate for meeting sexual needs, and one's personal appearance and self-esteem are related to their feelings of comfortable sexuality. Desiring sexual interaction is a healthy human desire, even in older adults.

54. d. Partial bed baths are generally given before breakfast due to incontinence to help the client feel comfortable and clean. Partial bed baths should include the genital and buttocks area since they are usually given because of incontinence.

55. a. The nurse aide should positively reinforce the resident's appropriate behavior, so smiling and rewarding her good behavior is the best action. Ignoring positive behavior does not help the patient to continue it, and teasing is not appropriate. The nurse aide should report to the nurse that the client has episodes of not swearing so that the nurse knows the plan is working.

56. b. Do not startle the resident, as this may agitate her. The aide should speak quietly as he enters the room. Suddenly turning on the light may startle the resident and increase her agitation, and an agitated client may interpret touch as a threat and lash out at the aide. Shouting can further agitate the client because it may make you appear to be aggressive.

57. b. Consideration of cultural or religious beliefs is important to all patients. Clients should not be made to wait for their food for any reason, and the dietician should be called that day by the nurse to report the client's religious preferences. Clients should not be forced to do something that is against their religion.

58. c. The other answer choices do not address the resident's right to practice her religion. Religious preferences need to be considered in client care, even by physicians. Bacon is a pork product and thus inappropriate to serve this client. Healthy alternatives can be found for dietary needs.

59. c. Listening to someone shows that you are very interested in what he or she is saying.

60. c. Threatening to withhold activities and food is verbally abusive. Choice **a** is incorrect because this is an inappropriate restriction that can hinder rehabilitation. Choice **b** is incorrect because threats are not discipline. Choice **d** is incorrect because this is abusive behavior; however, there is no physical contact, thus this it is not physical abuse.

61. a. Always call for help first in an emergency. The aide should call for help first, before he takes any physical action. Abdominal thrusts are not used until the rescuer verifies that the client's airway is blocked.

62. d. The first step for any lost belongings is always to notify the charge nurse. The nurse should report their loss before looking for them. The nurse aide does not report directly to the administrator or to the physician.

63. b. Nursing assistants work under the supervision of practical and registered nurses and perform tasks assigned them. Choice **a** is incorrect; nurse aides can participate in planning client care, but they are not responsible for it. Choice **c** is incorrect; all personnel should ask for help when needed, including nurse aides. Choice **d** is incorrect; nurse aides should focus on their own assignments and not be concerned about the assignments of others.

64. c. A nurse aide should answer any call light as soon as possible. Choice **a** is incorrect; nurse aides are responsible to answer call lights for all clients, when in a position to do so. Choice **b** is incorrect; clients should not be made to feel that they need to wait in line for care, even when it is busy. Choice **d** is incorrect; the nurse aide should answer the call light as soon as possible to assure that there is not an emergency.

65. b. Placing the client in a side-lying position prevents aspiration of the vomitus. Choice **a** is incorrect; while the nurse aide does need to clean the client, this is not the priority. Choice **c** is incorrect; the client is lying down and thus cannot use an emesis basin. Choice **d** incorrect; the nurse aide should call the charge nurse after he places the client on her side.

66. c. You should follow the clean-to-dirty principle, with the meatus considered cleaner than the catheter tubing. Choice **a** is incorrect; washing toward the meatus drags bacteria up the catheter into the meatus, possibly causing infection. Choice **b** is incorrect; soap and water should be used in catheter care. Choice **d** incorrect; alcohol can cause irritation of the urinary mucosa.

67. c. Applying restraints without an order or without consent can be considered *false imprisonment*. Choice **a** is incorrect because *slander* is transient, usually verbal, defamation of character. Choice **b** is incorrect because *battery* is unlawful physical contact. Choice **d** is incorrect because *negligence* is failure to exercise reasonable care.

68. b. H.S. is the medical abbreviation for hours of sleep. Choice **a** is incorrect; the medical abbreviation for before meals is a.c. Choice **c** is incorrect; the medical abbreviation for after meals is p.c. Choice **d** is incorrect; while not commonly used, o.m. means on morning.

69. d. Of the choices listed, only choice **d** contains a soft diet. Choices **a**, **b**, and **c** all contain foods difficult to eat without teeth.

70. a. If the client does not want to talk about death, the family should be allowed to talk privately, away from the client. Choices **b** and **d** are incorrect because the client's wishes should be respected and clients should not be forced to talk about something they do not want to talk about. Choice **c** is incorrect; the family should be able to verbalize their feelings now and not have to wait.

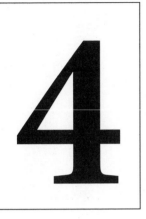

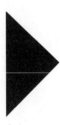

NURSING ASSISTANT/NURSE AIDE PRACTICE EXAM 2

CHAPTER SUMMARY

This is the second of five practice exams in this book based on the National Nurse Aide Assessment Program (NNAAP) written exam. This exam will give you more practice with the kinds of questions you are likely to see on the exam.

Like the first exam in this book, the exam in this chapter follows the NNAAP exam for certified nursing assistants. Now that you have taken one exam, you should be more comfortable with the format. If you followed the advice of this book and went back to your training materials to brush up on the areas you had trouble with in the first exam, you will probably do better on the second exam.

When you finish the exam, check your answers against the answer key that follows the exam. Read the explanations carefully; they will help you see why you missed the questions you did. You can also use the explanations to help you brush up on areas that give you trouble. Then refer to the chart in the Appendix (page 159) to see which kinds of questions were the most difficult for you. You should also go back to review your training materials and textbook, focusing on these areas in particular, before you take the third practice exam.

Practice Exam 2

	a	b	c	d			a	b	c	d			a	b	c	d
1.	ⓐ	ⓑ	ⓒ	ⓓ		26.	ⓐ	ⓑ	ⓒ	ⓓ		51.	ⓐ	ⓑ	ⓒ	ⓓ
2.	ⓐ	ⓑ	ⓒ	ⓓ		27.	ⓐ	ⓑ	ⓒ	ⓓ		52.	ⓐ	ⓑ	ⓒ	ⓓ
3.	ⓐ	ⓑ	ⓒ	ⓓ		28.	ⓐ	ⓑ	ⓒ	ⓓ		53.	ⓐ	ⓑ	ⓒ	ⓓ
4.	ⓐ	ⓑ	ⓒ	ⓓ		29.	ⓐ	ⓑ	ⓒ	ⓓ		54.	ⓐ	ⓑ	ⓒ	ⓓ
5.	ⓐ	ⓑ	ⓒ	ⓓ		30.	ⓐ	ⓑ	ⓒ	ⓓ		55.	ⓐ	ⓑ	ⓒ	ⓓ
6.	ⓐ	ⓑ	ⓒ	ⓓ		31.	ⓐ	ⓑ	ⓒ	ⓓ		56.	ⓐ	ⓑ	ⓒ	ⓓ
7.	ⓐ	ⓑ	ⓒ	ⓓ		32.	ⓐ	ⓑ	ⓒ	ⓓ		57.	ⓐ	ⓑ	ⓒ	ⓓ
8.	ⓐ	ⓑ	ⓒ	ⓓ		33.	ⓐ	ⓑ	ⓒ	ⓓ		58.	ⓐ	ⓑ	ⓒ	ⓓ
9.	ⓐ	ⓑ	ⓒ	ⓓ		34.	ⓐ	ⓑ	ⓒ	ⓓ		59.	ⓐ	ⓑ	ⓒ	ⓓ
10.	ⓐ	ⓑ	ⓒ	ⓓ		35.	ⓐ	ⓑ	ⓒ	ⓓ		60.	ⓐ	ⓑ	ⓒ	ⓓ
11.	ⓐ	ⓑ	ⓒ	ⓓ		36.	ⓐ	ⓑ	ⓒ	ⓓ		61.	ⓐ	ⓑ	ⓒ	ⓓ
12.	ⓐ	ⓑ	ⓒ	ⓓ		37.	ⓐ	ⓑ	ⓒ	ⓓ		62.	ⓐ	ⓑ	ⓒ	ⓓ
13.	ⓐ	ⓑ	ⓒ	ⓓ		38.	ⓐ	ⓑ	ⓒ	ⓓ		63.	ⓐ	ⓑ	ⓒ	ⓓ
14.	ⓐ	ⓑ	ⓒ	ⓓ		39.	ⓐ	ⓑ	ⓒ	ⓓ		64.	ⓐ	ⓑ	ⓒ	ⓓ
15.	ⓐ	ⓑ	ⓒ	ⓓ		40.	ⓐ	ⓑ	ⓒ	ⓓ		65.	ⓐ	ⓑ	ⓒ	ⓓ
16.	ⓐ	ⓑ	ⓒ	ⓓ		41.	ⓐ	ⓑ	ⓒ	ⓓ		66.	ⓐ	ⓑ	ⓒ	ⓓ
17.	ⓐ	ⓑ	ⓒ	ⓓ		42.	ⓐ	ⓑ	ⓒ	ⓓ		67.	ⓐ	ⓑ	ⓒ	ⓓ
18.	ⓐ	ⓑ	ⓒ	ⓓ		43.	ⓐ	ⓑ	ⓒ	ⓓ		68.	ⓐ	ⓑ	ⓒ	ⓓ
19.	ⓐ	ⓑ	ⓒ	ⓓ		44.	ⓐ	ⓑ	ⓒ	ⓓ		69.	ⓐ	ⓑ	ⓒ	ⓓ
20.	ⓐ	ⓑ	ⓒ	ⓓ		45.	ⓐ	ⓑ	ⓒ	ⓓ		70.	ⓐ	ⓑ	ⓒ	ⓓ
21.	ⓐ	ⓑ	ⓒ	ⓓ		46.	ⓐ	ⓑ	ⓒ	ⓓ						
22.	ⓐ	ⓑ	ⓒ	ⓓ		47.	ⓐ	ⓑ	ⓒ	ⓓ						
23.	ⓐ	ⓑ	ⓒ	ⓓ		48.	ⓐ	ⓑ	ⓒ	ⓓ						
24.	ⓐ	ⓑ	ⓒ	ⓓ		49.	ⓐ	ⓑ	ⓒ	ⓓ						
25.	ⓐ	ⓑ	ⓒ	ⓓ		50.	ⓐ	ⓑ	ⓒ	ⓓ						

Practice Exam 2

1. When should postmortem care be performed?
  a. after the family views the body
  b. immediately after the doctor pronounces the patient dead
  c. when rigor mortis sets in
  d. after the body goes to the morgue

2. A walker may be used if the client can
  a. support some weight.
  b. use her hands well.
  c. balance without help.
  d. walk independently.

3. A cane should be used on
  a. the affected (weak) side of the body.
  b. the unaffected (strong) side of the body.
  c. the side with the strongest arm.
  d. the weak side one day, and the strong side the next day.

4. A nurse aide is collecting linens for a bed change and drops a sheet on the floor. What should the nurse aide do?
  a. Ignore it and leave it on the floor.
  b. Place it back on the linen cart.
  c. Discard it in the soiled linen hamper.
  d. Use it anyway.

5. When applying a cold treatment to a patient, it is important to observe the patient closely for signs of
  a. redness.
  b. dizziness.
  c. fainting.
  d. cyanosis.

6. The purpose of correctly positioning the client is to
  a. prevent skin breakdown.
  b. maintain function of joints and muscles.
  c. increase comfort.
  d. all of the above

7. A surgical bed should be left in what position?
  a. Fowler's position
  b. lowest horizontal position
  c. semi-Fowler's position
  d. level with the stretcher

8. The preferred way to remove a bedpan from a client who is unable to lift her buttocks is to
  a. use a mechanical lifting device.
  b. have another nursing assistant lift the client.
  c. turn the client to the side while holding the pan.
  d. slowly slide the pan from under the client.

9. After shaving a patient with a safety razor, the nurse aide should
  a. cover it before discarding.
  b. wrap it in a paper towel and drop it into the trash can.
  c. dispose of it in a sharps container.
  d. place it in the patient's drawer for reuse.

10. When a client complains that his dentures are hurting, the appropriate action is to
  a. encourage him to wear the dentures more often.
  b. report the complaint to the charge nurse.
  c. report the complaint to the physician.
  d. put the dentures on the bedside table.

11. A nurse aide notices that a water pitcher has spilled onto the floor. The best action for the aide to perform is to
  a. wipe it up immediately.
  b. cover it with a towel.
  c. notify the charge nurse.
  d. contact housekeeping.

12. Upon entering a room, the nurse aide notices that a patient is not breathing. The aide's first action is to
  a. call for help.
  b. lay the patient down on his back.
  c. give four quick breaths.
  d. give ten abdominal thrusts.

13. A patient is on bed rest, wearing anti-embolitic stockings. How often should the stockings be removed?
  a. never
  b. q2h
  c. at least twice a day
  d. q6h

14. Pressure ulcers (decubitus ulcers) can be prevented by
  a. changing the client's position every two hours.
  b. placing a gel or foam pad on top of the mattress.
  c. increasing the client's consumption of vitamin C.
  d. both **a** and **b**

15. The first step in getting a client up to walk is to
  a. sit the client on the side of the bed.
  b. put the client's slippers on.
  c. check the activity order.
  d. tell the client that he will be getting up.

16. A client's vital signs are as follows: 118/80-98.8-80-30. Which finding should be reported at once?
  a. blood pressure
  b. temperature
  c. pulse
  d. respiration

17. All of the following can cause an inaccurate oral temperature reading EXCEPT
  a. drinking a hot cup of tea ten minutes before the reading.
  b. using an electronic thermometer.
  c. failing to shake down a glass thermometer.
  d. vigorous exercise prior to the reading.

18. Diastolic blood pressure is determined by
  a. listening for the first clear sound.
  b. listening for the last clear sound.
  c. subtracting the lower number from the top.
  d. adding the top and bottom numbers.

19. All of the following are correct when measuring blood pressure, EXCEPT
  a. do not assess blood pressure in an arm with an IV running.
  b. do not take the blood pressure in the same arm as where a person had a mastectomy.
  c. use the biggest cuff possible to get an accurate reading.
  d. make sure the room is quiet so you can hear before taking blood pressures.

20. The first step in performing any procedure is to
  a. explain the procedure.
  b. gather needed equipment.
  c. perform proper handwashing.
  d. provide privacy.

21. Which of the following best destroys all bacteria?
   a. soaking in alcohol
   b. washing with bleach
   c. sterilizing
   d. scrubbing in hot water

22. In the event of a fire in a client's room, the nurse aide should first
   a. notify the charge nurse.
   b. turn on a fire alarm.
   c. get the client to a safe place.
   d. use a fire extinguisher.

23. Safe use of oxygen therapy includes
   a. always setting the flow meter at 2–3 liters per minute.
   b. using wool blankets only.
   c. cleansing the nasal prongs each shift with alcohol.
   d. posting a "no smoking" sign on the door.

24. During CPR, the client should be lying
   a. flat on a hard surface.
   b. with head and shoulders elevated.
   c. with feet raised on a pillow.
   d. flat on the bed to prevent injuries.

25. A procedure manual is a
   a. written set of instructions on how to perform procedures.
   b. set of directions needed to complete a nurse aide's job description.
   c. book of directions for administering medications.
   d. book listing the procedures a nurse aide has been assigned to do.

26. If a client cannot speak English, the nurse aide should
   a. have the family interpret.
   b. ask the charge nurse to arrange for an interpreter.
   c. call the doctor to talk to the client.
   d. tell the client that she cannot answer the question.

27. The accepted way to identify a client is to
   a. check the bed name and number.
   b. check the identification band.
   c. ask the client's name.
   d. call the client by name.

28. Which of the following best describes nail care?
   a. Nail care is not needed for the elderly.
   b. Use scissors for all nail care.
   c. All clients need nail care.
   d. Check with the charge nurse for nail care instructions.

29. When performing perineal care on a male client, always
   a. clean the scrotum first.
   b. retract the foreskin if uncircumcised.
   c. clean from front to back.
   d. hold the penis at a 90-degree angle.

30. Back rubs aid in all of the following EXCEPT
   a. improving posture.
   b. improving circulation.
   c. increasing one-to-one interaction.
   d. relaxing the client.

31. A client's elbows are dry and red. The nurse aide should
   a. report this to the charge nurse.
   b. apply lotion to the elbows.
   c. apply elbow protectors.
   d. perform range of motion exercises.

32. A decubitus ulcer can be caused by all of the
following EXCEPT
   a. poor nutrition.
   b. pressure on the skin.
   c. poor circulation.
   d. cotton clothing.

33. The nursing assistant shampoos a client's hair
to improve all of the following EXCEPT
   a. circulation to the client's scalp.
   b. the client's general appearance.
   c. the client's sense of well-being.
   d. the rate of the client's hair growth.

34. When removing a soiled gown from a client
who has an IV, the best action is to
   a. remove the opposite arm from the gown
   first.
   b. have the nurse remove the IV needle.
   c. disconnect the bag and tubing.
   d. slip the gown over the IV solution bag.

35. If a client does not eat all the food on his tray,
the first thing an aide should do is
   a. notify the charge nurse.
   b. ask the client why he has not finished.
   c. remove the tray.
   d. urge the client to eat all the food.

36. The client states that a mistake has been made:
There is salt on her tray, although the doctor
has ordered a low-salt diet. The nurse aide
should
   a. explain this means no salt when preparing
   food.
   b. tell the client not to use the salt.
   c. check the diet order with the charge nurse.
   d. call the kitchen for a new tray.

37. Which of the following provides identification
of clients in long-term care facilities?
   a. identification bracelet
   b. photograph
   c. identification bracelet and photograph
   d. calling clients by name

38. Before transferring a client from the bed to a
wheelchair, the nurse aide should sit her on the
edge of the bed for a few minutes to
   a. rearrange her gown or clothing.
   b. prevent orthostatic hypotension.
   c. position and secure the wheelchair.
   d. rest and remove the transfer belt.

39. The client's religion forbids eating meat. Beef
stew is being served for lunch. The nurse aide
should
   a. tell the client to eat it because she needs
   protein.
   b. tell the client it is all right since her doctor
   ordered the diet.
   c. ask the nurse to call the kitchen.
   d. tell the client that religious restrictions are
   not as important as her health.

40. It is important to remember that dying patients
   a. have the same needs for care as other
   patients.
   b. need to be by themselves in a quiet room.
   c. do not need to be consulted regarding their
   care.
   d. are usually in pain.

41. Dying patients and their families
   a. always pass through five stages of dying in
   order.
   b. always accept death before it occurs.
   c. may go back and forth among the five stages.
   d. must go through all stages of dying before
   they die.

42. Which of the following is an early sign of dementia in an elderly client?
 a. refusing to eat a meal
 b. not knowing who she is
 c. frequent urination
 d. complaining of headaches

43. Clients with Alzheimer's disease may have all of the following characteristics EXCEPT
 a. physical wasting away.
 b. memory loss.
 c. wandering.
 d. irritability.

44. When a client turns on the call light every few minutes, the appropriate response is to
 a. ask the client not to call so often.
 b. stop by the room more often.
 c. place the call light out of reach.
 d. tell the client how busy the staff is.

45. The doctor writes an order for "do not resuscitate" (DNR). What does this mean?
 a. Put the client on a machine if she stops breathing.
 b. The client needs to be kept alive.
 c. CPR will not be performed.
 d. Start CPR immediately if the client stops breathing.

46. How a client reacts to illness and disability is most dependent on his
 a. age and stage of life.
 b. spouse's support.
 c. income and level of education.
 d. support system and life history.

47. A client with dementia makes sexual advances toward another client who has dementia. The nurse aide should
 a. allow it; OBRA '87 states that clients must be allowed to fulfill sexual needs.
 b. ask them to keep their sexual activity in a private place.
 c. ignore it so as not to embarrass them.
 d. tell the charge nurse, since a client with dementia is unable to give consent.

48. A client hits a nurse aide during lunch. The appropriate response is to
 a. call the charge nurse for help.
 b. continue to feed her.
 c. apply a restraint.
 d. yell at her to stop hitting.

49. A resident is confined to her bed. What might keep her from getting pressure sores?
 a. a plastic draw sheet
 b. a foot board
 c. body lotion
 d. an air mattress

50. If the client is in traction, the nurse aide should never
 a. monitor affected skin temperature.
 b. give a total bed bath.
 c. change the position of weights.
 d. monitor distal pulses.

51. Security for a client's dentures includes
 a. keeping them in a tissue in a dresser drawer.
 b. placing them in a labeled denture cup.
 c. insisting the resident wear the dentures.
 d. placing an identifying mark on the dentures.

52. If family members bring new clothes in for an ECF resident, the nurse aide should
   a. put them in the resident's dresser drawers.
   b. label them with the resident's name.
   c. ask the family to remove an equal number of old clothes.
   d. make sure the charge nurse sees the clothes.

53. The charge nurse instructs the nurse aide to clean an ECF resident's closet. The nurse aide should
   a. ask the family to do it.
   b. get another nurse aide to do it.
   c. enlist help from the client.
   d. have the client do it.

54. Before dressing an ECF resident, the nurse aide should
   a. check the order.
   b. choose the client's clothes.
   c. close the door.
   d. report to the charge nurse.

55. Confidentiality refers to
   a. never sharing client information.
   b. the client's right to privacy.
   c. not documenting information in the client's chart.
   d. the client's right to have insurance.

56. During A.M. care, the nurse aide nicks a resident while shaving him. What should she do first?
   a. Report it to the charge nurse.
   b. Do nothing.
   c. Apply pressure and stop the bleeding.
   d. Place a bandage on it.

57. Maintaining good interpersonal relationships depends on
   a. agreeing with the crowd.
   b. communicating clearly with others.
   c. following orders without question.
   d. avoiding contact after work hours.

58. If a nursing assistant does not know how to complete an assignment, he should
   a. ask another nursing assistant.
   b. ask the client for his preference.
   c. contact the charge nurse for help.
   d. utilize a policy manual.

59. Reporting what the client tells you is an example of
   a. subjective observation.
   b. objective observation.
   c. primary observation.
   d. secondary observation.

60. Incontinence means that the patient is
   a. unable to make decisions.
   b. unable to speak.
   c. experiencing a disorder that comes with aging.
   d. in need of medical attention.

61. Failure to raise the side rails on the bed of a confused client is an act of
   a. malpractice.
   b. negligence.
   c. overt commission.
   d. breaking a criminal law.

62. During a job interview, it is important to tell the interviewer about
   a. qualifications.
   b. childcare needs.
   c. scheduling problems.
   d. salary expectations.

63. When a nurse aide cannot work due to illness, the nurse aide should
   a. arrange for someone to cover his or her shift.
   b. contact the supervisor as soon as possible.
   c. call the charge nurse one hour before the shift begins.
   d. wait until the charge nurse calls to find out where the aide is.

64. What is the main goal of OBRA '87?
   a. to provide a safe environment for residents of extended-care and hospice facilities
   b. to provide prompt payment of care costs for residents covered by Medicare and Medicaid
   c. to make sure that healthcare providers meet the requirements nationwide by passing a competency and skill test to provide quality care
   d. to shorten the hospital stay of patients who can be attended at home by a nurse aide

65. The client asks to see a priest. The nurse aide should
   a. ask the charge nurse to call a priest.
   b. tell the client to see if a priest walks by his or her door.
   c. call the doctor.
   d. tell the client to call herself.

66. When caring for a client who has just been placed on NPO, the nurse aide should first
   a. encourage the client not to think about food and water.
   b. encourage the client to eat and drink.
   c. remove the water pitcher and all items of food and drink.
   d. give the client meticulous mouth care.

67. If a nurse aide sees another employee hit a client, the nurse aide should
   a. tell the employee to stop.
   b. keep an eye out to see if it happens again.
   c. tell another nurse aide.
   d. report it to the charge nurse immediately.

68. Which statement about mouth care for unconscious residents is correct?
   a. Unconscious residents may be able to hear you speaking to them during mouth care.
   b. Unconscious residents can both swallow and spit.
   c. Unconscious residents do not need to be observed for mouth sores.
   d. Unconscious residents have very moist gum tissue.

69. A hearing-impaired client has the right to all of the following EXCEPT
   a. written notes.
   b. an interpreter.
   c. assistance with hearing aids.
   d. purchase of the most expensive hearing aid.

70. When documenting a client's vital signs, the nurse aide makes a mistake. The nurse aide should
   a. cover the mistake with heavy black marker.
   b. cover the mistake with correction fluid.
   c. make a single line over it, write "error" and initial it.
   d. ignore it.

Answers

1. b. Postmortem care needs to be done before rigor mortis sets in so that the patient's appearance can be maintained. Once rigor mortis sets in, the body will be difficult to position. Postmortem care should occur before the family comes to view the body to remove any bodily fluids and treatment remnants. In some facilities, the funeral director completes postmortem care; however it is initiated on the medical unit.

2. a. A resident must be able to support some weight before using a walker. Hand strength alone is not adequate for walker usage, and though balance is important, the patient must first be able to support some weight. If the person can walk independently, she does not need a walker.

3. b. If the cane is not used on the strong side, the resident may fall. Switching between sides will not strengthen the weak side, and the client may fall when the cane is used on the weak side. Choice **c** is incorrect because though arm strength is important, it is not as important as leg strength.

4. c. To prevent contamination and the spread of microorganisms, the sheet should be put in the soiled linen hamper. Linens act as fomites, and this linen has been contaminated and cannot be used until it is washed. Leaving bed linens on the floor creates a fall hazard.

5. d. Cyanosis is an indication of poor circulation, which could lead to tissue death. The nurse aide should stop the treatment and report it to the charge nurse. Redness would be an issue with hot treatment, not with cold treatment. Cold packs should not result in dizziness or fainting.

6. d. Correctly positioning a patient should prevent skin breakdown, increase comfort, and maintain the function of joints and muscles.

7. d. The bed should be level with the stretcher. This makes a transfer safe. Choice **a** is incorrect; in Fowler's position, the head of the bed is raised between 45 and 60 degrees, making transfer from the stretcher difficult and unsafe. Choice **b** is incorrect; the lowest position will not be level with the stretcher, making transfer unsafe. Choice **c** is incorrect; in semi-Fowler's position, the head of the bed is raised between 30 and 45 degrees, making transfer from the stretcher difficult and unsafe.

8. c. Turning the resident is the easiest method, and it is important to hold the pan to prevent spilling the contents. Choice **a** is incorrect; mechanical lifts are used for people who are very heavy or who are unable to assist in the transfer. Choice **b** is incorrect; having another aide assist in lifting the patient is a possible way, but not the preferred way since that help may not be available when needed and you do not want the client to sit on the bedpan any longer than necessary. Choice **d** is incorrect; slowly sliding the pan from under the client risks the possibility of spilling the contents into the bed.

9. c. Sharps containers are puncture resistant. They are used to prevent contact with bloodborne pathogens. Sharps should never be tossed into the trash. They may cause injury, and there is concern of serious infection. Safety razors are for one-time use.

10. b. Always bring such complaints to the charge nurse. Choice **a** is incorrect; poorly fitting dentures are painful and can cause injury to the mouth. Choice **c** is incorrect; the nurse aide reports directly to the nurse, not the physician. Choice **d** is incorrect; dentures are kept safely in a denture cup, labeled with the client's name. Leaving them on the table risks both contamination and damage.

11. a. Take care of spills immediately, or a patient may be injured while waiting for housekeeping. It is not necessary to notify the charge nurse for this, and leaving the spill to go find the charge nurse or housekeeping increases the chance of someone falling on it. Covering it with a towel could create a fall hazard.

12. a. Call for help to activate the facility's emergency medical services. Early activation increases the client's chances for survival. Choice **b** is a correct action, but not the first action. Choices **c** and **d** are incorrect; check the airway before giving rescue breaths and do not start thrusts until you verify the person's airway is obstructed.

13. c. To allow normal blood flow to the lower extremities, the stockings should be removed twice a day. Anti-embolism stockings are removed every 8 to 12 hours to allow for adequate circulation. They prevent blood from pooling in the lower extremities, and therefore should not be removed too often.

14. d. Changing position frequently and using a gel or foam pad are both key. There is no data to suggest that vitamin C prevents pressure ulcers.

15. c. Always make sure the resident is allowed to get up first. The nurse does sit the client on the side of the bed before standing, put the client's slippers on before standing, and tell the client that he will be getting up, but not before checking the activity order.

16. d. The respiratory rate of the client is elevated. The blood pressure, temperature, and pulse are within normal limits.

17. b. Electronic thermometers are commonly used for assessing temperature. Drinking hot liquids, failing to shake down a glass thermometer, and exercising vigorously prior to an oral temperature reading cause an inaccurate reading.

18. b. The diastolic blood pressure occurs when the heart muscle relaxes. It is the bottom number of the reading and is the last sound heard before silence. The systolic blood pressure occurs when the heart muscle contracts, and the difference between the systolic and diastolic pressure is the pulse pressure. There is no reason to add the systolic and diastolic pressures.

19. c. Always use a cuff that fits. If the cuff is too large, you will get a reading that is too low. Choice **a** is incorrect; inflating the cuff may cause pain at the IV site and may cause the IV catheter to dislodge. Choice **b** is incorrect; some people who have had mastectomies also have had axillary (armpit) lymph nodes removed, which disrupts fluid flow in the arm and can lead to an inaccurate blood pressure reading. Choice **d** is incorrect; blood pressure may be difficult to hear, and thus the room should be quiet.

20. c. Infection control (handwashing) is always the first step in a procedure. Explaining the procedure is important and assuring privacy is important, but you should wash your hands before approaching the client. Wash your hands before touching equipment to avoid contamination.

21. c. Sterilization is the most thorough method of destroying bacteria. Antiseptics, such as alcohol, are used to prevent pathogens from spreading and may kill them. Disinfectants, such as bleach, can kill bacteria, but are too strong to use on the skin. Sanitation, including scrubbing in hot water, removes pathogens to prevent them from spreading.

22. c. Always get the client to safety first. Do not use time to notify the nurse. Turn on the alarm after getting the client to safety. You can use the fire extinguisher in the event of a small fire, but do so after getting the client to safety.

23. d. Smoking in bed brings all three elements of a fire together: linens for fuel, heat from the cigarette, and oxygen from the air. Choice **a** is incorrect, because the flow is determined by the physician. Choice **b** is incorrect, because wool can cause sparks. Choice **c** is incorrect, because alcohol causes drying.

24. a. The client should be lying flat on a hard surface to assure adequate compression and blood flow. The head and shoulders should be level with the rest of the body, and the feet should be level with the rest of the body. A bed mattress is too soft for effective chest compressions.

25. a. A procedure manual is a written set of instructions on how to perform procedures. A job description contains the general tasks, or functions, and responsibilities of that position. The procedure for administering medications would probably be found in the procedure manual, but the procedure manual would contain other procedures. The nurse aide assignments will most likely be created by the charge nurse.

26. b. It is mandatory to provide a certified interpreter to clients not fluent in English. Choice **a** is incorrect; using a family member to interpret sacrifices confidentiality. Choice **c** is incorrect; this is not appropriate for either translation or the nurse aide role. Choice **d** is incorrect; clients have a right to have their questions answered as quickly as possible.

27. b. An identification band is the only definitive way to identify the patient. A confused patient may answer to any name or may not know his name. A confused client may also be in the wrong bed.

28. c. All residents need nail care, and nail care is part of the nurse aide role. The nursing assistant should be able to obtain information needed from the care plan. Nails are cut with nail clippers.

29. b. Material may build up under the foreskin in uncircumcised males unless the foreskin is retracted for cleaning. Choices **a**, **b**, and **c** are incorrect. You should wash the penis before the scrotum, move from the tip of the penis to the base, and hold the penis slightly away from the body.

30. a. Back rubs are not used to improve posture. They improve circulation, give the nurse aide some time to talk to the client, and help to relax the client.

31. a. Report this to the charge nurse, since there are many reasons for redness. The redness and dryness may not be due to dry skin or friction rubbing. Range of motion may cause additional problems, depending on the cause of the redness and dryness.

32. d. Poor circulation, poor nutrition, and pressure on the skin all can cause decubitus ulcer. Poor circulation is a risk factor for pressure ulcers because the skin is already deprived of nutrients and oxygen. Poor nutrition is a risk factor for pressure ulcers. Pressure deprives the skin of blood flow and thus nutrients and oxygen, causing cells to die.

33. d. Shampooing can improve circulation to the client's scalp, the client's appearance, and the client's sense of well-being, but not hair growth rate.

34. a. Remove the sleeve from the arm without tubing first. The IV catheter is not removed for clothing changes, and the IV is not disconnected by the nurse aide.

35. b. The patient may not be eating due to personal dislike of the food. Asking first allows the nurse aide to request a replacement if the problem is simple. Notifying the charge nurse is not the first thing the nurse aide should do. You should remove the tray after trying to find out why the client will not eat. The client may simply need more seasoning. Do not force clients to eat.

36. c. Any diet question must be answered before the resident eats. The nurse aide should not conduct dietary teaching, and should always check the diet order with the nurse first.

37. c. Both identification bracelets *and* photographs are used for identification purposes in long-term care facilities. Confused clients may not know their own names.

38. b. *Orthostatic hypotension* is the light-headed feeling we all get when we rise too quickly. The gown or clothing is rearranged once the client is in the wheelchair, and the wheelchair should be positioned and secured before moving the client. The transfer belt is not removed before moving the client.

39. c. The other answers do not address the resident's right to practice religion or her right to choice. Religious restrictions are to be respected by healthcare providers.

40. a. Not all dying patients have the same problems, but they have all the same care needs as anyone else. Choice **b** is incorrect; many dying patients want companionship in their final hours. Choice **c** is incorrect; dying patients should be consulted regarding their care needs. Choice **d** is incorrect; not all dying patients are in pain.

41. c. Because each dying resident has unique emotional needs, each person will go through the stages at different times and in a different order. We now know that people experience loss differently and that they may not experience all the stages, nor may they experience them in order. Many people do not accept death before it occurs.

42. b. Memory loss is a sign of dementia. Refusal to eat is not a sign of dementia, but difficulty cooking a meal is an early sign. Headaches and frequent urination are not signs of dementia.

43. a. Clients with Alzheimer's disease should not have signs of physical wasting away, unless they have not been cared for. This may be a sign of neglect. Memory loss, wandering, and irritability are characteristic of Alzheimer's disease.

44. b. Patients who use their call bell frequently are usually afraid they will be ignored if they don't often call. Stopping in frequently reassures them. The client should always have access to the call bell. Asking the client to not call so often is inappropriate, and telling the client the staff is busy can increase her fear that her needs will not be met.

45. c. "Do not resuscitate" means that no attempts will be made to resuscitate the patient. Ventilators will not be used if there is a DNR order and the patient will not be kept alive artificially. CPR should not be initiated.

46. d. A person's total environment always affects everything that person does and thinks. Age and stage of life do affect a client's reactions, but they are not the most critical factors. A patient's overall support system plays a stronger role than just the spouse's support. Income and level of education do affect a client's reactions, but they are not the most critical factors.

47. d. Clients with dementia are not able to give consent; therefore, the nurse aide has a responsibility to protect clients from sexual advances. Choice **a** is incorrect; while OBRA '87 does state that clients must be allowed to fulfill their sexual needs, clients with dementia cannot legally consent to sexual activity. Choices **b** and **c** are incorrect; this is inappropriate sexual activity because clients with dementia cannot legally consent to sexual activity.

48. a. Obtaining assistance is the only correct way to deal with abuse by a resident. This is abusive behavior, and it should not be ignored. Choice **c** is incorrect, because restraints require physician's orders. Choice **d** is incorrect; yelling at patients is also abusive.

49. d. An air mattress relieves pressure. Air pressure alteration reduces pressure against the body to prevent circulation impairment. Choice **a** is incorrect; a plastic draw sheet can irritate delicate skin by holding moisture against the skin. Choice **b** is incorrect; a foot board is helpful, but alone will not prevent pressure sores. Choice **c** is incorrect; lotion and massage are helpful, but will not prevent pressure sores alone.

50. c. Position of weights in traction is ordered by the physician. Therefore, the nursing assistant should never change the position of the weights without an order. The skin temperature should be monitored because coolness can indicate decreased circulation. Total bed baths are not contraindicated because of traction. Distal pulses should be monitored in clients with traction to check for adequate circulation.

51. b. Every resident with dentures must have a labeled denture cup to ensure security of costly dentures. Residents should not be forced to wear their dentures, and markers and pens should not be used on dentures.

52. b. All residents have the right to their own personal possessions. Labels allow the aide to better provide protection. Choice **a** is incorrect; the nurse aide should label the clothing before placing them in the resident's dresser. Choice **c** is incorrect; the resident is entitled to keep her personal possessions. Choice **d** is incorrect; the nurse aide can label and store clothing without consulting the nurse.

53. c. The client has a legal right to decide what to keep and what to throw away, but may need assistance in the cleaning process. The family is not required to clean the resident's closets, and the nurse aide should not pass off her responsibilities to another nurse aide. ECF clients are not usually well enough to clean their closets, nor should they be expected to clean them.

54. c. A nurse aide should always close the door to promote privacy. Except for unusual circumstances, there are no orders for how a client should be dressed, and dressing does not require reporting to the charge nurse. The client has the right to choose her own clothing.

55. b. Confidentiality refers to the client's right to privacy. Choice **a** is incorrect; client information is shared with the rest of the healthcare team on the client's hospital or ECF unit. Choice **c** is incorrect; chart documentation is important to promote communication and to provide a lasting document of the client's hospitalization or ECF stay. Choice **d** is incorrect; clients do not have a right to insurance.

56. c. The first step is to stop the bleeding in order to ensure the patient's comfort. Choice **a** is incorrect; the nurse aide should report this to the charge nurse, but it is not the priority. Choice **b** is incorrect; doing nothing can cause excessive bleeding in clients who have bleeding tendencies, such as those who are taking anti-clotting medications, and may also lead to infection. Choice **d** is incorrect; bleeding should be stopped first.

57. b. Clear communication is critical to good interpersonal relationships, while contact avoidance can damage them. One can disagree and still maintain good interpersonal relationships. Following orders without questioning can lead to resentment and doing things improperly if the orders are not correct.

58. c. Asking for help from a supervisor is a critical component to career growth. Choice **a** is incorrect; the other nursing assistant may also not know how to complete the assignment. Choice **b** is incorrect; nurse aides should not ask clients for assistance with understanding assignments. Choice **d** is incorrect; policy manuals contain policies, not assignment procedures.

59. a. Subjective observation comes from what the client tells you. Objective observation comes from what you see, hear, feel, or smell. Primary observation relates to what should be considered first. Secondary observation relates to what is considered after primary observation.

60. d. Incontinence is generally due to a medical problem. It is important to adhere to a bowel/bladder training program. *Aboulia* is the term for the inability to make decisions. *Aphasic* is the term for the inability to speak. *Gero* and *geri* are used in terms that relate to aging.

61. b. Negligence is an unintentional act of injury. It is breech of a civil law, not criminal law. Malpractice is negligent treatment of a patient by a professional. Overt commission means openly acting on something, such as deliberately injuring a patient.

62. a. You need to sell yourself during the interview. Ask about benefits and your personal needs after you get the job. Do not discuss scheduling problems until after you have been offered the position, and do not discuss salary expectations until after you have been offered the position or at least until the interviewer has discussed it with you.

63. b. Contact a supervisor as soon as possible, so that a replacement can be found in a timely manner. Choice **a** is incorrect; the nurse aide is not responsible to cover his or her shift. Choice **c** is incorrect; calling one hour before the shift begins decreases the chance that someone else can be found to cover it. Choice **d** is incorrect; waiting for the charge nurse to call you is not responsible behavior and may result in disciplinary action.

64. c. All healthcare providers must be responsible for their actions. OBRA '87 does not cover hospice facilities, oversee payment of care costs, or act to shorten hospital stays.

65. a. It is a client's right to have clergy available as requested. The client should not have to rely on chance to see a clergy person, nor should she have to contact the clergy person herself. It is not the physician's duty to call the priest in this case.

66. c. NPO means nothing by mouth, so removing all food and water will reduce temptations. Encouraging someone to not think about something typically results in her thinking about it. The client had just been placed on NPO and thus mouth care is not required at this time.

67. d. Tell the charge nurse immediately when you suspect abuse. You are legally obligated to report it, and you want to do so as soon as possible to prevent further abuse. The nurse aide should not directly confront an abusive employee, nor should she wait to see if it will happen again, as that can result in another client being injured. Answer **c** is also incorrect; another nurse aide cannot do anything to help, so you should tell the charge nurse.

68. a. The last sense to leave is hearing; speak with kindness and be aware of what you say. Unconscious residents cannot swallow and spit, which means mouth care must be carried out carefully to prevent aspiration. The mouth and lips of an unconscious patient can easily become dry and sore, thus they need frequent mouth care and observation for sores.

69. d. The client has the right to assistance with hearing aids, but there is no right that pertains to getting expensive options. A hearing-impaired client may need written notes to understand procedures and directions or an interpreter, especially if the client uses sign language.

70. c. Charting errors are corrected by using a single black line through the error, marking it with the word "error," and initialing it. The client's chart is a legal document, and covering the error with a heavy black marker or correction fluid is unacceptable.

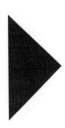

5 ▶ NURSING ASSISTANT/NURSE AIDE PRACTICE EXAM 3

CHAPTER SUMMARY

This is the third of five practice exams in this book based on the National Nurse Aide Assessment Program (NNAAP) written exam. Use this test to identify which types of questions are still giving you problems.

Y ou are now beginning to be very familiar with the format of the nursing assistant exam. Your practice test-taking experience will help you most, however, if you have created a situation as close as possible to the real one.

For this third exam, simulate taking the real test. Find a quiet place where you will not be disturbed. Have several sharpened pencils and a good eraser nearby. Complete the test in one sitting, setting a timer or a stopwatch. You should have plenty of time to answer all of the questions when you take the real exam, but you want to work quickly without rushing.

As before, the answer sheet you should use is on the next page. Following the exam is an answer key, with all the answers explained. These explanations will help you see where you need to concentrate further study. Once you have reviewed the answer explanations and referred to the question-type breakdown in the Appendix (page 159), you will know which parts of your training materials you need to concentrate on before you take the fourth exam.

Practice Exam 3

1.	ⓐ	ⓑ	ⓒ	ⓓ
2.	ⓐ	ⓑ	ⓒ	ⓓ
3.	ⓐ	ⓑ	ⓒ	ⓓ
4.	ⓐ	ⓑ	ⓒ	ⓓ
5.	ⓐ	ⓑ	ⓒ	ⓓ
6.	ⓐ	ⓑ	ⓒ	ⓓ
7.	ⓐ	ⓑ	ⓒ	ⓓ
8.	ⓐ	ⓑ	ⓒ	ⓓ
9.	ⓐ	ⓑ	ⓒ	ⓓ
10.	ⓐ	ⓑ	ⓒ	ⓓ
11.	ⓐ	ⓑ	ⓒ	ⓓ
12.	ⓐ	ⓑ	ⓒ	ⓓ
13.	ⓐ	ⓑ	ⓒ	ⓓ
14.	ⓐ	ⓑ	ⓒ	ⓓ
15.	ⓐ	ⓑ	ⓒ	ⓓ
16.	ⓐ	ⓑ	ⓒ	ⓓ
17.	ⓐ	ⓑ	ⓒ	ⓓ
18.	ⓐ	ⓑ	ⓒ	ⓓ
19.	ⓐ	ⓑ	ⓒ	ⓓ
20.	ⓐ	ⓑ	ⓒ	ⓓ
21.	ⓐ	ⓑ	ⓒ	ⓓ
22.	ⓐ	ⓑ	ⓒ	ⓓ
23.	ⓐ	ⓑ	ⓒ	ⓓ
24.	ⓐ	ⓑ	ⓒ	ⓓ
25.	ⓐ	ⓑ	ⓒ	ⓓ

26.	ⓐ	ⓑ	ⓒ	ⓓ
27.	ⓐ	ⓑ	ⓒ	ⓓ
28.	ⓐ	ⓑ	ⓒ	ⓓ
29.	ⓐ	ⓑ	ⓒ	ⓓ
30.	ⓐ	ⓑ	ⓒ	ⓓ
31.	ⓐ	ⓑ	ⓒ	ⓓ
32.	ⓐ	ⓑ	ⓒ	ⓓ
33.	ⓐ	ⓑ	ⓒ	ⓓ
34.	ⓐ	ⓑ	ⓒ	ⓓ
35.	ⓐ	ⓑ	ⓒ	ⓓ
36.	ⓐ	ⓑ	ⓒ	ⓓ
37.	ⓐ	ⓑ	ⓒ	ⓓ
38.	ⓐ	ⓑ	ⓒ	ⓓ
39.	ⓐ	ⓑ	ⓒ	ⓓ
40.	ⓐ	ⓑ	ⓒ	ⓓ
41.	ⓐ	ⓑ	ⓒ	ⓓ
42.	ⓐ	ⓑ	ⓒ	ⓓ
43.	ⓐ	ⓑ	ⓒ	ⓓ
44.	ⓐ	ⓑ	ⓒ	ⓓ
45.	ⓐ	ⓑ	ⓒ	ⓓ
46.	ⓐ	ⓑ	ⓒ	ⓓ
47.	ⓐ	ⓑ	ⓒ	ⓓ
48.	ⓐ	ⓑ	ⓒ	ⓓ
49.	ⓐ	ⓑ	ⓒ	ⓓ
50.	ⓐ	ⓑ	ⓒ	ⓓ

51.	ⓐ	ⓑ	ⓒ	ⓓ
52.	ⓐ	ⓑ	ⓒ	ⓓ
53.	ⓐ	ⓑ	ⓒ	ⓓ
54.	ⓐ	ⓑ	ⓒ	ⓓ
55.	ⓐ	ⓑ	ⓒ	ⓓ
56.	ⓐ	ⓑ	ⓒ	ⓓ
57.	ⓐ	ⓑ	ⓒ	ⓓ
58.	ⓐ	ⓑ	ⓒ	ⓓ
59.	ⓐ	ⓑ	ⓒ	ⓓ
60.	ⓐ	ⓑ	ⓒ	ⓓ
61.	ⓐ	ⓑ	ⓒ	ⓓ
62.	ⓐ	ⓑ	ⓒ	ⓓ
63.	ⓐ	ⓑ	ⓒ	ⓓ
64.	ⓐ	ⓑ	ⓒ	ⓓ
65.	ⓐ	ⓑ	ⓒ	ⓓ
66.	ⓐ	ⓑ	ⓒ	ⓓ
67.	ⓐ	ⓑ	ⓒ	ⓓ
68.	ⓐ	ⓑ	ⓒ	ⓓ
69.	ⓐ	ⓑ	ⓒ	ⓓ
70.	ⓐ	ⓑ	ⓒ	ⓓ

Practice Exam 3

1. Inactivity and immobility may cause all of the following EXCEPT
   a. pressure ulcers.
   b. permanent contractures.
   c. increased intestinal peristalsis.
   d. secretions remaining in the lungs.

2. The nurse aide knows that the term "up ad lib" means the client
   a. is not permitted out of bed.
   b. is independent with balanced periods of rest and activity.
   c. is out of bed at mealtime only.
   d. will need assistance for all activities of daily living.

3. When lifting a patient, it is important to use good body mechanics. The nurse aide should
   a. keep the patient at arm's length.
   b. bend at the knees.
   c. twist at the waist.
   d. move the patient rapidly.

4. A common sign of approaching death is
   a. increased appetite.
   b. normal or elevated vital signs.
   c. severe, unceasing pain.
   d. decreased body functions.

5. Tuberculosis is a disease of the
   a. throat.
   b. colon.
   c. lungs.
   d. kidney.

6. The nursing assistant notes that a client's respiratory rate is zero. The nursing assistant should
   a. resume the client's normal care.
   b. wait ten minutes and check the client's respirations again.
   c. inform the client's family that the client is dead.
   d. contact the charge nurse immediately.

7. After a client dies, the client's spouse wishes to share his emotions. The nurse aide should
   a. listen and try to provide comfort.
   b. change the subject.
   c. tell the spouse to contact a counselor.
   d. send him to the charge nurse.

8. An example of a special device to help prevent contractures is a(n)
   a. handroll.
   b. doppler.
   c. air mattress.
   d. manometer.

9. Falsely stating that a coworker took a client's money is an example of
   a. negligence.
   b. assault.
   c. defamation.
   d. hoarding.

10. Hemiplegia refers to
   a. paralysis on one side of the body.
   b. paralysis of both legs.
   c. paralysis of both arms.
   d. paralysis of all four extremities.

11. The most accurate method of measuring body temperature is
a. rectal.
b. oral.
c. axial.
d. feeling the forehead.

12. Which of the following sets of vital signs should be reported immediately?
a. T–98.6, P–60, R–14, BP–120/60
b. T–102.4, P–100, R–32, BP–180/100
c. T–99.6, P–80, R–16, BP–132/70
d. T–97.6, P–82, R–20, BP–110/60

13. A client consumed 180 cc of tea, 60 cc of soup and 120 cc of ice cream. What is her total fluid intake?
a. 180 cc
b. 240 cc
c. 360 cc
d. 400 cc

14. A client is placed on strict I&O after surgery. The nurse aide should
a. keep the client NPO.
b. record the client's entire solid food intake.
c. record the client's fluid intake only.
d. record the client's fluid intake and urine output.

15. Which of the following would be included in a client's output record?
a. urine, food eaten, and IV solutions
b. urine, emesis, and bleeding
c. liquids taken in during the shift
d. bowel movements only

16. Which of the following is an intake-and-output problem that the nurse aide must report?
a. The client states that he is not hungry.
b. The client requests a bedpan.
c. The client has not voided in eight hours.
d. The client's eight-hour output is 600 cc.

17. A client's water pitcher holds 500 cc. The pitcher is full at the beginning of the shift, and empty halfway through the shift. The nurse refills it, and the client drinks half of the pitcher by the end of the shift. The total water intake for this client at the end of the shift is
a. 250 cc.
b. 500 cc.
c. 750 cc.
d. 1,000 cc.

18. The nurse aide finds a damaged piece of equipment. The nurse aide should
a. dispose of it immediately.
b. use it until new equipment arrives.
c. report it immediately.
d. repair it herself and then use it.

19. After caring for a confused client, the nurse aide fails to pull up the safety rails, and the client falls out of the bed and fractures a hip. This is called
a. abuse.
b. negligence.
c. battery.
d. assault.

20. A nursing assistant is giving foot care to a resident. What should he NOT do?
a. Remove corns.
b. Soak the resident's feet in warm water.
c. Check for skin breakdown.
d. Clean under the toenails using an orangewood stick.

21. When restraints are in use, the nurse aide should report all of the following EXCEPT
   a. the type of device being used.
   b. the time the restraint was released.
   c. unusual observations about the client's skin.
   d. the aide's experience with restraints.

22. The pulse located in the neck is called the
   a. apical pulse.
   b. femoral pulse.
   c. radial pulse.
   d. carotid pulse.

23. A client complains of numbness on one side of the body. The client's grip is weak and speech is slurred. The nurse aide should
   a. call the doctor because the client had a CVA.
   b. check the blood pressure to verify it is a CVA.
   c. check the client later to see if it may be a CVA.
   d. report it to the charge nurse immediately because it may be a CVA.

24. When providing perineal care to a female patient, it is important to wash from the front to the back to avoid spreading bacteria found in the resident's
   a. pancreas.
   b. vulvus.
   c. meatus.
   d. rectum.

25. The order "vital signs q.i.d." means to record vital signs
   a. four times per day.
   b. twice per day.
   c. morning and evening.
   d. once per shift.

26. The nurse aide notices that a client has an open red area on her coccyx that is draining. The nurse aide should
   a. wash the area with soap and water and apply alcohol.
   b. ask another nursing assistant to look at it and give his opinion.
   c. check it again at the same time the next day.
   d. tell the charge nurse so she can check it.

27. A nursing assistant is ambulating a client in the hallway. Suddenly, the client complains of chest pain and shortness of breath. The nurse aid should first
   a. walk the client back to the client's bed immediately.
   b. get the sphygmomanometer and take the client's blood pressure.
   c. stay with the client and call for help.
   d. help the client to the floor and go find a phone to call 911.

28. A client finishes drinking a glass of cold water just as the nurse aide arrives to take the client's rectal temperature. The nurse aide should
   a. wait 15 minutes before taking the temperature.
   b. give the client some warm water to counter the effect of the cold.
   c. report this to the charge nurse.
   d. take the client's rectal temperature as planned.

29. Which of the following observations should be reported immediately?
   a. T–98.2, P–88, R–20
   b. yellow-colored urine
   c. bluish tint to lips and skin
   d. skin that is warm and dry to the touch

30. Microorganisms can be spread by direct and indirect contact. An example of *indirect contact* is
   a. bathing the patient.
   b. using contaminated blood.
   c. touching objects or dirty instruments.
   d. breathing dust particles in the air.

31. Which statement about handwashing is correct?
   a. The faucet is clean and may be touched when washing hands.
   b. Wash at least two inches above the wrist.
   c. Hands can be washed in any temperature water.
   d. Hand sanitizers never substitute for handwashing.

32. The nursing assistant finds a client lying on the floor. The nursing assistant should first
   a. run out of the room and get help.
   b. help her up into a chair.
   c. gently shake her and ask if she is okay.
   d. call 911.

33. Which statement about use of fire extinguishers is correct?
   a. Any fire extinguisher can be used on any fire.
   b. Each extinguisher should be used for the correct type of fire.
   c. Nurse aides are not responsible for using fire extinguishers.
   d. Fire extinguishers should not be used for small fires.

34. A client begins to choke during feeding. The client is conscious but unable to speak or cough. The nurse aide should
   a. shake the client and ask if the client is okay.
   b. call the physician.
   c. administer abdominal thrusts.
   d. sweep one finger in the client's mouth to check for obstruction.

35. The nurse aide should tell the licensed nurse if a patient with _____ does not finish the food on his tray.
   a. stroke
   b. cancer
   c. diabetes
   d. Alzheimer's disease

36. Which of the following tasks is NOT within the job description of the nurse aide?
   a. providing the resident with ROM
   b. shaving the resident
   c. applying a sterile dressing to an open wound
   d. recording vital signs

37. Giving good oral care to a client includes all of the following except
   a. wearing gloves.
   b. handling and storing dentures carefully.
   c. using dental floss.
   d. removing oxygen before brushing.

38. To prevent infection in a client with an indwelling catheter, the nurse aide should
   a. keep the drainage bag higher than the bladder.
   b. do perineal care from front to back as needed.
   c. let the tubing make a U loop below the bed.
   d. do perineal care every other night.

39. A client is on a clear fluid diet. The client's lunch tray may consist of
    a. tea, broth, and gelatin.
    b. coffee, milk and soup.
    c. milk, soup and ice cream.
    d. coffee, broth and crackers.

40. Which statement about injuries to clients and staff members is correct?
    a. Injuries should be treated and reported on an incident report.
    b. Injuries to staff can be ignored if they are minor.
    c. Injuries should be reported only if they are major.
    d. Injuries should be treated but do not need to be reported.

41. Lying on a job application is an example of
    a. tort.
    b. malpractice.
    c. fraud.
    d. negligence.

42. While shaving a client, the nurse aide accidentally nicks the client. The nurse aide should
    a. put alcohol on the nick.
    b. report it to the charge nurse.
    c. report it to the physician.
    d. ignore it, since it is just a nick.

43. When witnessing another aide hitting an irritable client, the nurse aide should
    a. tell the aide to stop.
    b. observe the aide for a few days.
    c. report it to the charge nurse.
    d. ignore it; the client is irritable.

44. When clients are in a healthcare institution, they can expect their treatment to conform to the
    a. Infection Control Manual.
    b. Patient's Bill of Rights.
    c. Policy and Procedure Manual.
    d. Physician's Code of Ethics.

45. A conversation about a client in the hospital's elevator violates the
    a. client's right to privacy.
    b. client's right to medical care.
    c. client's right to review his records.
    d. client's right to ask questions.

46. A client constantly makes sexual remarks to staff. When discussing this at a team meeting, the administration decides to instruct staff to call the client by name and tell the client,
    a. "You are making me blush."
    b. "Your comments are not acceptable."
    c. "You are quite a character."
    d. "You should be ashamed of yourself."

47. Which of the five senses would best detect a rash?
    a. sight
    b. smell
    c. touch
    d. hearing

48. The best way a nurse aide can clean an infant's eyes is with a(n)
    a. cotton swab lubricated with petroleum jelly.
    b. moist cotton ball, wiping from the inner to the outer corner.
    c. alcohol wipe, using circular motions.
    d. hot towel, wiping from the outer to the inner corner.

49. A client who is hard of hearing repeatedly turns her light on. When responding to this client's call light, the nurse aide should
   a. listen carefully to determine her needs.
   b. talk loudly over the intercom so that she can hear.
   c. train her to use the call light less often.
   d. tell the charge nurse that the client is attention seeking.

50. Another employee asks the nurse aide what is wrong with a newly admitted client. What should the nurse aide do?
   a. Tell the employee, since information can be shared with coworkers.
   b. Discuss the situation with the charge nurse before talking to the other employee.
   c. Wait until break time to discuss the client with the other employee.
   d. Tell the other employee that aides are not allowed to talk about the clients.

51. Most hospital stays are
   a. one week.
   b. a few days.
   c. two days.
   d. as long as necessary.

52. When caring for a female client, how should the nurse aide address her?
   a. "Ma'am"
   b. "Miss"
   c. by her first name
   d. by her surname

53. A client is on a low-sodium diet. The nurse aide notes that the client received bacon on the breakfast tray. The nurse aide should
   a. remove the bacon from the tray.
   b. instruct the client not to eat the bacon.
   c. take the breakfast tray to the charge nurse.
   d. take the breakfast tray back to the dietician.

54. While providing personal care for a client, the nurse aide should
   a. uncover the client completely so that she can work quickly.
   b. uncover only the area she is working on.
   c. keep the client completely covered and work under the covers.
   d. leave the curtain open at all times.

55. When providing morning (A.M.) care for the client, the nurse aide should
   a. let the client do as much as he is able to.
   b. do everything for the client so it is done correctly.
   c. care only for clients who are the same sex.
   d. work as quickly as possible.

56. A client with left-sided weakness should be taught to
   a. put his right arm into his shirt first.
   b. put his left arm into his shirt first.
   c. put both arms in the shirt at the same time.
   d. wear a hospital gown to make dressing easier.

57. It is important not to shake linens to prevent the spread of what type of microorganisms?
   a. bacteria
   b. fungi
   c. rickettsiae
   d. fomites

58. If a client objects to certain food for religious or cultural reasons, the nurse aide should
   a. tell him to consult with his doctor.
   b. offer to get something different for him.
   c. tell him he will have to speak to the dietician tomorrow.
   d. tell him he will be given a tube feeding if he won't eat.

59. A terminally ill resident refuses his bath and throws a water basin across the room. Which stage of dying does this behavior represent?
a. denial
b. anger
c. bargaining
d. acceptance

60. A terminally ill resident begs, "Please just let me live long enough to see my granddaughter." Which state of dying does this behavior represent?
a. denial
b. anger
c. bargaining
d. acceptance

61. An important thing the nurse aide can do for a dying client is to
a. leave her alone to allow for privacy.
b. give physical and emotional support.
c. encourage her to believe that a miracle may occur.
d. force her to eat three meals a day to keep up her strength.

62. What is most important to show the client in his new room?
a. the television remote control
b. how to lower and raise the bed
c. the location of the call bell and how to use it
d. where to store personal belongings

63. The older adult likes to feel positive about herself by sharing past achievements and experiences. The best way the nurse aide can encourage this is by
a. pairing the older adult with another talkative resident.
b. encouraging frequent rest periods to save energy for socializing.
c. listening to the older adult's past experiences.
d. telling the older adult that aides are too busy to listen to stories.

64. When caring for a client who is anxious, the nurse aide should do all of the following EXCEPT
a. remain calm.
b. make the client stay still.
c. provide a quiet atmosphere.
d. use simple, easy to understand words.

65. A client asks the nurse aide if she could have a few minutes to pray before her bath. The best response by the nurse aide would be to
a. tell her that her bath comes first.
b. allow her some private time to pray.
c. tell her to wait until clergy visits.
d. start bathing her.

66. During orientation to a new job, a nursing assistant realizes that the work shift ends at 3:30 P.M. and not 3:00 P.M. as previously thought. The nursing assistant's child needs to be picked up every day at 3:15 P.M. The nursing assistant should
a. discuss this with the charge nurse as soon as possible.
b. ask another nursing assistant to cover after 3:00 P.M.
c. leave early, as no one is likely to notice.
d. come in 15 minutes earlier in the morning.

67. The best definition of a certified nursing assistant is a
   a. graduate nurse who is registered and licensed by the state to practice nursing.
   b. licensed person who provides education about special diets.
   c. person who transcribes the physician's orders for patient care.
   d. person who is certified to give care under the direct supervision of a registered or licensed practical nurse.

68. When the nurse aide shows genuine interest and concern for the client, this is an example of
   a. honesty.
   b. caring.
   c. teamwork.
   d. accuracy.

69. When giving a bed bath, the nurse aide should
   a. put the bed in the low position.
   b. cover the resident with a bath blanket.
   c. wash the perineal area from back to front.
   d. place dirty towels and linens on the floor.

70. An indwelling catheter drains the bladder of
   a. feces.
   b. emesis.
   c. urine.
   d. blood.

Answers

1. c. Intestinal peristalsis decreases with inactivity and immobility. Pressure ulcers are the most common complication of immobility. Contractures occur when a joint is left in the same position for a long time, and decreased filling of the lungs from immobility allows fluid and mucous to build up in the lungs.

2. b. "Up ad lib" is an activity order suggesting the client can perform ADLs independently with periods of rest as needed. "Complete bed rest (CBR)" means that the client is not permitted out of bed. Clients allowed out of bed for mealtime only usually have an order that specifies this. "Ambulate with assistance" is the term usually used for clients who need assistance with activities.

3. b. It is important to use the large muscles in the legs and thighs to prevent back injury. Keeping the patient at arm's length risks the patient falling and the nurse aide hurting his back, and twisting at the waist can cause back strain. Moving the patient rapidly can cause injury to both the patient and the nurse aide.

4. d. As circulation slows, body functions decrease. Appetite and vital signs decrease when death approaches. Not all dying patients are in severe, unceasing pain.

5. c. Tuberculosis most commonly affects the lungs. A person with tuberculosis in the lungs can spread it to others through droplets in respiratory secretions. Tuberculosis does not usually affect the throat or colon. While it may spread to the kidneys, it is primarily a lung disorder.

6. d. A respiratory rate of zero may signal approaching death; contact the nurse immediately. Choice **a** is incorrect; a respiratory rate of zero means that the client is not breathing, and this should be reported immediately. Choice **b** is incorrect; the client will die if there is no immediate intervention—ten minutes is too long to wait. Choice **c** is incorrect; it is not the nurse aide's responsibility to notify the family when there is a death.

7. a. Caring for the family is part of the job, and thus the nurse aide should comfort the spouse. Nurse aides do not need to call the charge nurse; they can use their therapeutic communication skills to communicate with family and relatives of dying clients. If the client wants to share his emotions, the nurse aide should be a good listener and not change the subject.

8. a. A handroll is placed in the palm of the hand to prevent the hands and fingers from contracting into a flexed position. A doppler is a type of measuring device, such as an ultrasound or blood pressure device. An air mattress is used to prevent pressure ulcers. A manometer is an instrument used for measuring the pressure of gases and vapors.

9. c. *Defamation* is harming a person's reputation by words that you say (slander) or write (libel) intentionally. *Negligence* is a failure to exercise reasonable care; it is an unintentional wrong. *Assault* is threatening a person or attempting to touch a person without their consent. *Hoarding* is the accumulation of food and other items.

10. a. *Hemiplegia* refers to paralysis of one side of the body. *Paraplegia* refers to paralysis of the legs or lower body. *Cruciate paralysis* is paralysis of an upper extremity. *Quadriplegia* refers to paralysis of all four extremities.

11. a. The rectal temperature method is considered the most accurate, as the thermometer is in direct contact with membranes. An oral temperature reading can be affected by many factors, including the client's drinking hot or cold fluids just before the readings. The axillary temperature can be affected if the patient just washed under her arms or applied deodorant. Feeling the forehead is an inaccurate way to measure temperature; however, there are temporal thermometers that are swept across the head to measure temperature.

12. b. A temperature of 102.4°F is elevated. The patient's pulse indicates tachycardia, which is a fast pulse, and the patient's blood pressure is high, indicating hypertension. Choice **a** is incorrect; these vital signs are within normal limits. Choice **c** is incorrect; the temperature is at the high end of normal, as is the systolic blood pressure. These do need to be reported, but not immediately. Choice **d** is incorrect; these vital signs are within normal limits.

13. c. Ice cream is a fluid, so the client's total intake is 360 cc. 180 plus 60, plus 120, equals 360. Choice **a**, **b**, and **d** are incorrect because the numbers do not add up to 360.

14. d. I&O refers to fluid intake and urinary output, as well as other outputs, including drainage. Choice **a** is incorrect; the nurse aide cannot place a client on NPO without an order. Choice **b** is incorrect; solid food intake is not included in the I&O. Choice **c** is incorrect; this is only partially correct since fluids and output would be measured.

15. b. Urine, emesis, and bleeding are all considered output. Choice **a** is incorrect; food eaten is not included in I&O and IV solutions are included in the intake. Choice **c** is incorrect; liquids are part of the intake. Choice **d** is incorrect; bowel movements are included if liquid, but are not the only inclusion in output.

16. c. Failure to void (urinate) may indicate kidney failure. The normal adult urinary output is 1,500 cc per day, or approximately 500 cc per eight-hour shift. While a client's stating he is not hungry is important to note, this is not an I&O problem. A client's request for a bedpan is not typically reported.

17. c. A full water pitcher at 500 cc, plus a half pitcher at 250 cc equals 750 cc of water. 250 cc would be one half of the water pitcher. 500 cc would be a full water pitcher. 1,000 cc would be two full water pitchers.

18. c. Immediately reporting equipment damage can prevent an accident. It is not the nurse aide's role to repair equipment. Most equipment is costly and repairable, and thus should not be thrown away unless the nurse aide is told to do so. Using faulty equipment is hazardous and can result in injury.

19. b. *Negligence* is an unintentional wrong. *Abuse* is an intentional act that causes harm to another person. *Battery* is the infliction of injury. *Assault* is threatening a person or attempting to touch a person without his consent.

20. a. Only a podiatrist or a nurse can remove corns. Choice **b** is incorrect; soaking the feet may help to soften corns. Choice **c** is incorrect; the nurse aide should check the skin for signs of breakdown when performing foot care. Choice **d** is incorrect; an orangewood stick is used to clean underneath a person's toenails.

21. d. The aide's experience is not part of the client's record. There are different types of restraints, and thus the nurse aide should document the type used for the client. Restraints are removed every two hours to allow for repositioning, and can sometimes cause bruising and other complications. Both pieces of information should be recorded.

22. d. The *carotid pulse* is located in the neck. The *apical pulse* is located on the chest, over the apex of the heart. The *femoral pulse* is located in the groin area. The *radial pulse* is located on the inside of the wrist.

23. d. These are all signs of a possible CVA (stroke), and the nurse aide should report this to the charge nurse immediately to prevent further damage to the client. Choice **a** is incorrect; the client may be having a CVA, but it is not the nurse aide's role to call the physician. Choice **b** is incorrect; a CVA needs immediate medical attention, thus the nurse aide should not waste time taking the client's blood pressure. Choice **c** is incorrect; a CVA requires immediate attention, and thus the nurse aide needs to report these signs immediately.

24. d. Bacteria from the rectum can cause urinary tract infections. The pancreas is an internal organ located in the abdomen. Proper perineal care is used to prevent contaminating the vulvus or meatus with bacteria.

25. a. Q.i.d. means four times a day. B.i.d. means twice a day. Q.a.m. and q.p.m. mean every morning and evening. Qshift means once per shift.

26. d. An opening in the skin predisposes the client to infection and must be checked by the nurse. The nurse aide should not touch the area before telling the nurse, and alcohol would cause pain on an open wound. The wound may get worse if the nurse aide waits another day.

27. c. Do not leave the client in an emergency. Chest pain and dizziness may signal a myocardial infarction (heart attack). Choice **a** is incorrect; the client may be having a heart attack (myocardial infarction) and should not continue to ambulate. The nurse aide should not leave the client, so all other choices are incorrect.

28. d. Take the client's rectal temperature as planned, because the cool water would affect the oral, not rectal reading. Choice **a** is incorrect, because waiting 15 minutes after a client drinks cold water is for oral temperatures. Choice **b** is not necessary, since the nurse aide is taking a rectal temperature. Choice **c** is incorrect; there is no need to report this to the charge nurse.

29. c. Bluish discoloration (cyanosis) indicates low oxygen level in the body. The condition can be life threatening. T–98.2, P–88, R–20 are normal vital signs. Yellow is a normal color for urine. The skin should be warm and dry to the touch.

30. c. Objects such as bed linens, dishes, and dirty instruments harbor microorganisms. Bathing a patient, using contaminated blood, and breathing dust particles are all examples of direct contact.

31. b. Hands should be washed at least two inches above the wrist. Choice **a** is incorrect; the faucet is most likely contaminated by dirty hands. Choice **c** is incorrect; hands should be washed in warm water. Choice **d** is incorrect; according to the CDC, hand sanitizers can be used for routine hand decontamination.

32. c. Shaking and shouting helps determine if the client is conscious and oriented. Choice **a** is incorrect; the nurse aide should not leave the client. Choice **b** is incorrect; the client may be unconscious or not breathing. Choice **d** is incorrect; the nurse should first check the client, and then summon help. Calling 911 is not typical in an inpatient facility.

33. b. Different extinguishers are used on various types of fires. Choice **a** is incorrect; fires are classified as A (fueled by ordinary material), B (fueled by a petroleum product), or C (an electrical fire), and only ABC fire extinguishers can be used for all three. Choice **c** is incorrect; nurse aides are responsible for using fire extinguishers correctly. Choice **d** is incorrect; fire extinguishers are used for fires of all sizes.

34. c. Abdominal thrusts can dislodge the obstruction. Choice **a** is incorrect; the nurse aide witnessed the client choke during feeding and noted the client is unable to speak; therefore, the nurse aide knows the client is not okay and cannot respond to her. Choice **b** is incorrect; it is not the nurse aide's role to call a physician. Choice **d** is incorrect; sweeping the mouth may push the object further into the airway.

35. c. A diabetic's blood sugar is controlled by diet and medication. Any food not eaten will affect the blood sugar level. Missing part of one meal should not create problems for the client in situations **a**, **b**, or **d**. However, this should be reported at the end of the shift.

36. c. Only a licensed RN or LPN may perform sterile procedures. Nurse aides can perform range of motion exercises, as well as shave clients and record vital signs.

37. d. Oxygen does not interfere with oral hygiene. Gloves should be worn when performing oral care; dentures should be handled and stored correctly; and dental floss should be used when appropriate.

38. b. Always wipe from front to back to prevent rectal germs from entering the vagina or urinary tract. Keeping the drainage bag higher than the bladder can cause urine to back flow into the bladder, increasing the chance of infection. A U loop may also cause back flow to the bladder, increasing the risk for infection. Perineal care is performed at least daily.

39. a. Clear fluids are see-through. Milk, ice cream, coffee, and crackers are not clear fluids.

40. a. Minor and major injuries must be documented. Injuries to staff should never be ignored and should always be treated *and* reported.

41. c. *Fraud* denotes deception. A *tort* is a wrong that involves a breach of a civil duty. The Joint Commission defines *malpractice* as "improper or unethical conduct or unreasonable lack of skill by a holder of a professional or official position." The Joint Commission defines *negligence* as "failure to use such care as a reasonably prudent and careful person would use under similar circumstances."

42. b. Report it to the charge nurse; a nick can become infected, and all injuries must be reported immediately. Alcohol may sting, and nurse aides cannot apply alcohol without an order. The nurse aide does not report to the physician.

43. c. Abuse must be reported immediately. The nurse aide should not directly confront an abusive staff member, and waiting for a few days can risk the abuser injuring another client. Clients should never be hit, regardless of their behavior.

44. b. The Patient's Bill of Rights is a written statement that includes the rights clients are entitled to when receiving healthcare. The Infection Control Manual and the Policy and Procedure Manual do not address client treatment. The Physician Code of Ethics applies only to physicians.

45. a. Conversations regarding a client should never take place in a public area such as an elevator. This violates the client's rights to privacy. This situation does not violate the client's right to receive medical care, to review his records, or to ask questions.

46. b. The staff must tell the client that the behavior is inappropriate. Choice **a** is incorrect; this comment may increase the negative behavior if the client is trying to get a reaction from staff. Choice **c** is incorrect; this comment condones the behavior. Choice **d** is incorrect; this comment belittles the client.

47. a. Rashes are best detected by observation. Smell may be useful only if the rash is giving off an odor. Touch is only useful of the rash has a definite texture. Hearing is not useful in detecting a rash.

48. b. Infants' eyes are cleaned from inner to outer to prevent the spread of infection. A moist cotton ball is soft and will not injure the eye. Petroleum jelly is not a cleansing agent. Alcohol is not used to clean the eyes, and it can cause chemical damage to them. A hot towel can burn the delicate eyes, and wiping from outer to inner can increase the risk for infection.

49. a. Listening builds trust, and continuous call bell ringing may have an underlying reason, such as loneliness. Choice **b** is incorrect; a hearing-impaired person may not be able to understand the nurse aide over the call bell system, thus the nurse aide should respond in person. Choice **c** is incorrect; a client must have a way to communicate with staff at all times. Choice **d** is incorrect; the nurse aide should listen to the client to determine the client's needs.

50. d. The Patient's Bill of rights assures that clients' confidential information is shared only when necessary for care. The nurse aide should not discuss the client at any time with another employee, unless it is directly related to client care. Information is only shared with the immediate healthcare team as needed. The nurse aide should understand client confidentiality.

51. d. Hospital stays vary based on the patient's specific diagnosis and procedures. There is no one average hospital stay; the average length depends on the diagnosis.

52. d. Clients should be addressed by their surnames (e.g., Mrs. Smith). This shows that the aide respects the client's dignity. "Ma'am" is a term used by the military, not by hospital personnel, and "miss" may be viewed as condescending. Using a client's first name may be viewed as a sign of disrespect and should not be done unless requested by the client.

53. c. The client should not have the bacon. The charge nurse is responsible for contacting the dietician about the error. Choice **a** is incorrect; the client should not have the bacon, but there may be other inappropriate items on the tray. Choice **b** is incorrect; the client may eat it anyway. Choice **d** is incorrect; it is not the nurse aide's role to confer directly with the dietician.

54. b. Covering the areas of the body that the nurse aide is not working on will allow privacy and keep the body warm. Keeping the client uncovered deprives the client of her dignity, and also can cause discomfort from her being cold. Working under the covers makes care difficult and disallows the nurse aide to observe problems, such as skin redness. The curtain should remain closed, because the client has the right to privacy.

55. a. Encouraging independence allows clients to feel self-worth by participating in their own care. Choice **b** is incorrect; the nurse aide should foster independence and allow the client do as much as possible, even if not done correctly. Choice **c** is incorrect; in general, nurse aides care for clients of both genders; however some cultures require that care be given by persons of the same gender. Choice **d** is incorrect; care should not be rushed.

56. b. The client should put the weak arm in the shirt first. Putting the strong arm in first will make it difficult to finish putting on the shirt. It will be too difficult for the client to put both arms into the shirt at the same time. Clients should be encouraged to wear their own clothing to enhance self-esteem and normality.

57. d. Fomites are in or on some hospital equipment. Bacteria, fungi, and rickettsiae may be on fomites.

58. b. Consideration of cultural or religious beliefs is important to all clients. It is not usually necessary to call the physician for cultural preferences. However, if it becomes necessary, this should be handled by the nurse. The client is entitled to have a preferred food right away. However, the nurse aide should inform the nurse of the cultural preference so that the nurse can contact the dietician regarding future meals. Telling a client he will get a tube feeding if he will not eat is abusive behavior and may constitute assault because it is a threat.

59. b. The client is in the anger stage of dying, and the nurse aide should acknowledge the client's anger and allow him to talk about it. During denial, the resident will not believe that he is dying. During bargaining the resident hopes that he can somehow postpone death. During acceptance, the resident comes to terms with his mortality.

60. c. In bargaining, clients "want to make a deal" with someone who may be able to control their fate. The nurse should offer realistic support. During denial, the resident will not believe that he is dying. During anger, the client can be difficult and may act out his anger toward the staff. During acceptance, the resident comes to terms with his mortality.

61. b. Physical and emotional support are both vital to terminal clients. Choice **a** is incorrect; the dying client may not want to be alone. Choice **c** is incorrect; false hope is inappropriate. Choice **d** is incorrect; dying clients often lose their appetites and should not be forced to eat.

62. c. Providing a means to call a nurse is important to avoid injury and meet the client's needs. Choices **a**, **b**, and **d** are important, but not the most important things for the client to know.

63. c. Listening tells clients you are interested in what they have to say. Choice **a** is incorrect; this is helpful for socialization, but may not be the best way to promote positive feelings. Choice **b** is incorrect; this is helpful, but secondary. Choice **d** is incorrect; this is inappropriate, as nurse aides should listen to their clients.

64. b. Forcing an anxious client to stay still may increase the client's anxiety level. Your being calm will help the client to become calm, and a quiet environment assists in decreasing anxiety. Anxiety decreases cognition (thinking ability); therefore the nurse aide should speak in a calm, clear, easy-to-understand manner.

65. b. Respecting a client's spiritual needs is an important aspect of the client's care. A client's right to religious beliefs should be respected. Unless specifically requested, clients do not need clergy to pray. Choice **d** ignores both the client's religious beliefs and the client's right to be heard.

NURSING ASSISTANT/NURSE AIDE PRACTICE EXAM 3

66. a. Being honest and up front with your supervisor is the best approach. Choice **b** is incorrect; a nurse aide cannot ask another nurse aide to cover her work time. Choice **c** is incorrect; this is being dishonest and honesty is a critical quality for healthcare workers. Choice **d** is incorrect; the nurse aide cannot set her own hours; this requires making arrangements with the charge nurse or other appropriate personnel.

67. d. This is the only correct definition of a certified nursing assistant. The nursing assistant is always under the direct supervision of a licensed nurse. Choice **a** refers to a licensed nurse. Choice **b** refers to a licensed dietician. Choice **c** refers to a medical transcriber.

68. b. Nursing is caring. It is an attitude of interest and concern. *Honesty* is being truthful in one's words and actions. *Teamwork* is the ability to work well with others as a team. *Accuracy* is one's ability to do things correctly.

69. b. Privacy and warmth are in accordance with the Patient's Bill of Rights. Choice **a** is incorrect; when giving a bed bath, the nurse aide should place the bed in a high position to avoid injuring her back through constant bending. Choice **c** is incorrect; the perineal area is washed from front to back. Choice **d** is incorrect; dirty towels and linens are placed in the appropriate receptacle.

70. c. A catheter inserted in the bladder drains urine from the body.

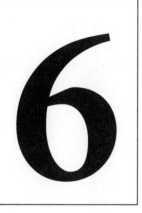

NURSING ASSISTANT/NURSE AIDE PRACTICE EXAM 4

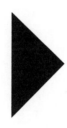

CHAPTER SUMMARY

This is the fourth of five practice exams in this book based on the National Nurse Aide Assessment Program (NNAAP) written exam. Use this test and the question breakdown in the Appendix (p. 159) to identify which types of questions are still giving you problems.

his is the second-to-the-last sample National Nurse Aide Assessment Program (NNAAP) written exam in this book. It is not any harder than the other three have been. It is simply another representation of what you might expect for the real test. Just as when you go to take the real test, there shouldn't be anything here to surprise you. That's the idea for the real test, too—that you won't be surprised, so you won't be unprepared. Check to see which test areas are still giving you trouble using the Appendix on page 159.

Practice Exam 4

1. ⓐ ⓑ ⓒ ⓓ
2. ⓐ ⓑ ⓒ ⓓ
3. ⓐ ⓑ ⓒ ⓓ
4. ⓐ ⓑ ⓒ ⓓ
5. ⓐ ⓑ ⓒ ⓓ
6. ⓐ ⓑ ⓒ ⓓ
7. ⓐ ⓑ ⓒ ⓓ
8. ⓐ ⓑ ⓒ ⓓ
9. ⓐ ⓑ ⓒ ⓓ
10. ⓐ ⓑ ⓒ ⓓ
11. ⓐ ⓑ ⓒ ⓓ
12. ⓐ ⓑ ⓒ ⓓ
13. ⓐ ⓑ ⓒ ⓓ
14. ⓐ ⓑ ⓒ ⓓ
15. ⓐ ⓑ ⓒ ⓓ
16. ⓐ ⓑ ⓒ ⓓ
17. ⓐ ⓑ ⓒ ⓓ
18. ⓐ ⓑ ⓒ ⓓ
19. ⓐ ⓑ ⓒ ⓓ
20. ⓐ ⓑ ⓒ ⓓ
21. ⓐ ⓑ ⓒ ⓓ
22. ⓐ ⓑ ⓒ ⓓ
23. ⓐ ⓑ ⓒ ⓓ
24. ⓐ ⓑ ⓒ ⓓ
25. ⓐ ⓑ ⓒ ⓓ
26. ⓐ ⓑ ⓒ ⓓ
27. ⓐ ⓑ ⓒ ⓓ
28. ⓐ ⓑ ⓒ ⓓ
29. ⓐ ⓑ ⓒ ⓓ
30. ⓐ ⓑ ⓒ ⓓ
31. ⓐ ⓑ ⓒ ⓓ
32. ⓐ ⓑ ⓒ ⓓ
33. ⓐ ⓑ ⓒ ⓓ
34. ⓐ ⓑ ⓒ ⓓ
35. ⓐ ⓑ ⓒ ⓓ
36. ⓐ ⓑ ⓒ ⓓ
37. ⓐ ⓑ ⓒ ⓓ
38. ⓐ ⓑ ⓒ ⓓ
39. ⓐ ⓑ ⓒ ⓓ
40. ⓐ ⓑ ⓒ ⓓ
41. ⓐ ⓑ ⓒ ⓓ
42. ⓐ ⓑ ⓒ ⓓ
43. ⓐ ⓑ ⓒ ⓓ
44. ⓐ ⓑ ⓒ ⓓ
45. ⓐ ⓑ ⓒ ⓓ
46. ⓐ ⓑ ⓒ ⓓ
47. ⓐ ⓑ ⓒ ⓓ
48. ⓐ ⓑ ⓒ ⓓ
49. ⓐ ⓑ ⓒ ⓓ
50. ⓐ ⓑ ⓒ ⓓ
51. ⓐ ⓑ ⓒ ⓓ
52. ⓐ ⓑ ⓒ ⓓ
53. ⓐ ⓑ ⓒ ⓓ
54. ⓐ ⓑ ⓒ ⓓ
55. ⓐ ⓑ ⓒ ⓓ
56. ⓐ ⓑ ⓒ ⓓ
57. ⓐ ⓑ ⓒ ⓓ
58. ⓐ ⓑ ⓒ ⓓ
59. ⓐ ⓑ ⓒ ⓓ
60. ⓐ ⓑ ⓒ ⓓ
61. ⓐ ⓑ ⓒ ⓓ
62. ⓐ ⓑ ⓒ ⓓ
63. ⓐ ⓑ ⓒ ⓓ
64. ⓐ ⓑ ⓒ ⓓ
65. ⓐ ⓑ ⓒ ⓓ
66. ⓐ ⓑ ⓒ ⓓ
67. ⓐ ⓑ ⓒ ⓓ
68. ⓐ ⓑ ⓒ ⓓ
69. ⓐ ⓑ ⓒ ⓓ
70. ⓐ ⓑ ⓒ ⓓ

Practice Exam 4

1. The charge nurse asks the nurse aide to place a client in the Fowler's position after the client eats breakfast. How should the aide position the client?
 a. lying with the head of the bed elevated at a 45- to 60-degree angle
 b. lying on the side with the knee and thigh drawn upward toward the chest
 c. lying flat on her side
 d. lying flat on her abdomen

2. How many stages of death were identified by Dr. Elizabeth Kübler-Ross?
 a. four
 b. five
 c. eight
 d. two

3. A cane should be used on
 a. the affected side.
 b. the unaffected side.
 c. either side, depending on how the client feels.
 d. the weak side one day and the strong side the next.

4. All of the following factors contribute to lack of appetite EXCEPT
 a. decreased activity.
 b. bad dentures.
 c. increased exercise.
 d. decreased saliva.

5. Atrophy is
 a. contracture.
 b. orthotic.
 c. muscle wasting.
 d. a fracture.

6. The nurse aide, a member of the healthcare team, can participate in many aspects of the nursing process, except for
 a. collecting data.
 b. planning the care.
 c. making observations.
 d. carrying out selected interventions.

7. When using crutches, the client's weight must rest on the
 a. armpit.
 b. knees.
 c. hand rests.
 d. shoulders.

8. How often should a client be repositioned if he cannot move himself?
 a. every hour
 b. every two hours
 c. every three hours
 d. every four hours

9. A client who had a CVA is going through a self-care/grooming program. The main goal of this program is for the client to
 a. be discharged sooner.
 b. gain independence.
 c. learn to accept the disability.
 d. improve his body image.

10. The goal of bladder training is to
 a. gain voluntary control of urination.
 b. stop using a catheter.
 c. prevent skin problems caused by incontinence.
 d. prevent urinary tract infections from indwelling catheters.

11. A resident sometimes chokes while eating. The nursing assistant should
   a. instruct his roommate to watch him eat.
   b. feed him to prevent problems.
   c. use the Heimlich maneuver between bites.
   d. observe him while he eats.

12. If a client complains of a burning, tingling area on her skin, the aide should first
   a. rub the area well with lotion.
   b. report the complaint to the licensed nurse.
   c. keep an eye on the area for a few days.
   d. use cornstarch on the area.

13. When changing a pillowcase, a nurse aide should not hold the pillow under his chin because this would
   a. tear the pillowcase.
   b. drop the pillowcase.
   c. dampen the pillowcase.
   d. spread bacteria.

14. A nonsterile dressing is one that is
   a. wet.
   b. dry.
   c. clean.
   d. new.

15. When asked to clean a resident's eye, the nurse aide should
   a. clean it from the outer corner to the inner corner.
   b. clean it with hydrogen peroxide.
   c. use a clean surface of the cloth each time he wipes.
   d. clean the eye with exudates first.

16. One nurse aide is assigned vital signs, while another is assigned bathing. This is an example of which type of nursing?
   a. primary
   b. patient-centered
   c. team
   d. modular

17. Gloves must be worn when
   a. providing pericare.
   b. making beds.
   c. washing a resident's hair.
   d. feeding a patient.

18. While the nurse aide was caring for a client for four hours, the client asked to be taken to the bathroom every 15 minutes. The nurse aide's best action is
   a. leaving the client on a padded bedpan.
   b. placing the client in bed with a waterproof underpad.
   c. giving the client some time to rest.
   d. discussing this with the charge nurse.

19. An elderly resident becomes confused and begins to wander. The nurse aide should
   a. restrain her to prevent injuries.
   b. orient her to time and place.
   c. tell her family about the behavior.
   d. report her behavior to the charge nurse.

20. The Hoyer lift is used for all of the following purposes EXCEPT
   a. preventing injuries to healthcare workers.
   b. supporting ambulatory clients.
   c. moving clients who are heavy.
   d. moving clients who are weak.

21. When performing active range-of-motion exercises for a resident, the nurse aide should
   a. move the joints until the resident feels pain.
   b. keep the body exposed to prevent overheating.
   c. have the client do as much as she can.
   d. minimize proper body mechanics.

22. Using a broad base of support means
   a. keeping the feet comfortably apart.
   b. keeping knees locked in place.
   c. holding objects away from the body.
   d. holding feet and hands as far from the body as possible.

23. If a client is in traction, the nursing assistant should NOT
   a. give a complete bed bath.
   b. monitor affected skin color.
   c. change the position of the weights.
   d. monitor all possible distal pulses.

24. When the nurse aide is moving the client up in bed, the pillow goes
   a. on the chair, out of the way.
   b. at the foot of the bed, out of the way.
   c. at the head of the bed, to protect the head.
   d. anywhere the client wants it.

25. Dangling a client's legs over the side of the bed is done to
   a. make sure she is able to sit up first.
   b. give her time to put on her shoes.
   c. prevent decubitus ulcers.
   d. prevent orthostatic hypotension.

26. Walking with a client is safest if done with a
   a. transfer belt.
   b. wheelchair a few steps behind him.
   c. Hoyer lift.
   d. nurse or doctor ready for emergencies.

27. When having a client sit up and dangle his legs before walking, the nurse aide should observe for all of the following EXCEPT
   a. cheerfulness.
   b. sudden paleness.
   c. excessive sweating.
   d. increased respirations.

28. When the nurse aide is transferring a client from the bed to the wheelchair, she should always
   a. unlock the brakes on the wheelchair.
   b. lock the brakes on the wheelchair first.
   c. use a Hoyer lift.
   d. put socks on the client first.

29. Before any transfer, the nurse aide should do all of the following EXCEPT
   a. have the nurse's approval.
   b. know the proper procedure.
   c. use a transfer belt if needed.
   d. check with the client's physician.

30. The pulse located in the wrist is called the
   a. carotid pulse.
   b. apical pulse.
   c. femoral pulse.
   d. radial pulse.

31. A patient is scheduled for an ECG. This stands for
   a. electroencephalogram.
   b. electrocardiogram.
   c. electroconvulsive therapy.
   d. electromyogram.

32. Which of the following sets of vital signs should be reported immediately?
   a. T–98.2 P–122 R–20 BP–84/40
   b. T–99.0 P–72 R–16 BP–134/82
   c. T–98.8 P–66 R–14 BP–100/62
   d. T–98.6 P–90 R–18 BP–120/70

33. A piece of linen that is placed beneath the client from shoulders to thighs is called
  a. an underpad.
  b. a spread.
  c. a drawsheet.
  d. a sheet.

34. Which bedmaking procedure is used when the client remains in the bed?
  a. occupied bedmaking procedure
  b. unoccupied bedmaking procedure
  c. circle bedmaking procedure
  d. procedure using only fitted sheets

35. Which complication may happen if a post-op client does not take in adequate fluids?
  a. constipation
  b. blood clots
  c. infection
  d. foot drop

36. Which type of client is most likely to have problems as a result of poor nail care?
  a. a cancer client
  b. a diabetic client
  c. a stroke client
  d. a developmentally disabled client

37. When performing mouth care for a client with right-sided weakness, the nurse aide should
  a. pay special attention to the left side of her mouth.
  b. let her do as much of it as she can.
  c. do the mouth care for her.
  d. tell her to do it herself.

38. A trochanter roll is used to
  a. keep the arm straight.
  b. keep the patient on the side.
  c. keep the hip in alignment.
  d. keep the leg flexed.

39. A resident with a paralyzed left arm may be able to feed herself if she uses a(n)
  a. plate guard.
  b. arm brace.
  c. sling.
  d. bib.

40. Which statement about residents with developmental disabilities is generally correct?
  a. They should be treated like children.
  b. They cannot walk or talk.
  c. They learn at a slower pace.
  d. They are suspicious of new people.

41. A diabetic client has had her leg amputated. Her need for sexuality will
  a. be more important for a while.
  b. be less important for a while.
  c. disappear forever.
  d. be unaffected.

42. Clients with Alzheimer's disease may show which of the following symptoms?
  a. high fever accompanied by chills
  b. clear memory of the recent and distant past
  c. chest pains and difficulty breathing
  d. physical and mental decline

43. If a client is upset and is yelling, the nurse aide should respond by
  a. saying sternly, "Quiet down!"
  b. offering to call her doctor.
  c. shutting her door for privacy.
  d. calmly sitting down with the client and listening.

44. A common sign of depression is
  a. attending activities daily.
  b. laughing and smiling.
  c. decreased appetite.
  d. socializing with friends.

45. A client who has just been told she is dying asks the nurse aide to help her make a list of things she wants to do before she dies. The nurse aide should
   a. tell her to wait for her family to help her.
   b. tell her that the list is not necessary.
   c. help her make the list.
   d. tell her not to worry because she has plenty of time.

46. To assist a client with his psychological needs, the nurse aide should
   a. be a good listener and show empathy.
   b. assure the client that everything will be okay.
   c. maintain the client's confidentiality.
   d. encourage the client to talk to his roommate.

47. A Catholic client refuses to eat meat on Fridays. Her lunch one Friday consists of a roast beef sandwich and a salad. The nurse aide should first
   a. tell the client to eat only the salad.
   b. offer to get her a meatless lunch.
   c. ask family members to bring in something else.
   d. request that a priest come and speak with her.

48. A nurse aide enters a room and finds a patient having sex with his wife. What should the nurse aide do?
   a. Ask him to stop.
   b. Step out of the room quietly and close the door.
   c. Report it to the charge nurse.
   d. Discuss it with another nurse aide.

49. A young, permanently handicapped resident tends to be very quiet and act as if nothing matters. The nurse aide can best show respect for her by
   a. including her in the plan of care.
   b. serving her dinner first.
   c. calling her by her first name.
   d. doing the client's care for her.

50. An example of using body language while communicating is
   a. using gestures and facial expressions.
   b. writing the message on paper.
   c. sharing your feelings and concerns.
   d. offering your advice and opinions.

51. A nurse aide smiles and nods her head while sitting with a client. This type of nonverbal communication best demonstrates
   a. encouragement for the client to continue talking.
   b. displeasure at having to listen to the client.
   c. agreement with everything that the client says.
   d. lack of available work for the nurse aide.

52. Barriers to effective communication include
   a. reflection.
   b. clarification.
   c. assuming.
   d. listening.

53. A client's best friend asks the nurse aide what is wrong with the client. The nurse aide's best response is
   a. "I'm sorry, I'm not allowed to discuss him with you."
   b. "You really should ask the charge nurse for that information."
   c. "I'll tell you, but keep it confidential."
   d. "I'm really not sure what is wrong with him."

54. A client who is alert and oriented refuses his bath. The best response from the nurse aide is
   a. "You must take a bath every day, even if you don't want to."
   b. "I doubt your roommate would appreciate the smell."
   c. "Can you tell me why you don't feel like bathing today?"
   d. "Is there something wrong with taking a bath?"

55. An example of false imprisonment is
   a. using restraints without a doctor's order or the client's consent.
   b. closing the door to the client's room.
   c. treating the client differently because of his religious beliefs.
   d. refusing to answer a call light that rings frequently.

56. Another nurse aide is not providing adequate care for the residents. The nurse aide who notices this should
   a. keep a list of activities not performed.
   b. tell all the other staff members.
   c. complete the inadequate care himself.
   d. report this to the charge nurse immediately.

57. A nurse aide notes a bright red rash on a client. This type of observation is termed
   a. subjective.
   b. objective.
   c. primary.
   d. secondary.

58. A former union leader was the victim of an industrial accident and is now a resident. To maintain this resident's dignity, the nurse aide may suggest that the client
   a. read industrial magazines.
   b. serve on the resident council.
   c. watch business-oriented movies.
   d. relax and play bingo.

59. A client's daughter wants to help with her mother's care. The nurse aide should
   a. allow her to do whatever care she wants to do.
   b. tell her she cannot perform any care for her mother.
   c. let her do the bathing and dressing only.
   d. have her do whatever the nurse agrees to.

60. It is important to remember that a client in the last stage of a terminal illness should
   a. be left alone to grieve.
   b. be offered care to meet her physical and emotional needs.
   c. be cared for only by relatives and close friends.
   d. not be offered any choices about her care.

61. Allowing clients to dress in their personal clothing
   a. decreases clothing costs.
   b. improves client well-being.
   c. makes it easier to dress clients.
   d. enhances infection control.

62. A young, postoperative client has his door closed, and the nurse aide needs to check his vital signs. The nurse aide should
   a. knock on the door and wait for the client to respond.
   b. assume he does not want to be disturbed and leave him alone.
   c. immediately open the door and walk in.
   d. knock and enter without need for a response.

63. A restraint may be used on a resident for
   a. discipline.
   b. staff convenience.
   c. roommate request.
   d. safety.

64. A client insists on wearing a striped blouse and plaid pants. The nurse aide should
   a. help her choose a more appropriate outfit.
   b. tell her that she will look uncoordinated.
   c. respect her clothing choice.
   d. select an outfit for her.

65. Failure to perform service for which a person is trained is called
   a. discrimination.
   b. malpractice.
   c. defamation.
   d. false imprisonment.

66. After assisting a client to the bedside commode, the nurse aide should
   a. leave the curtain open so she can see the client.
   b. provide privacy with the curtain pulled.
   c. make the client's bed while she is sitting on the commode.
   d. tell the client that she can use the commode only once a shift.

67. A healthcare team includes all of the following EXCEPT
   a. nurse aides.
   b. registered nurses.
   c. receptionists.
   d. physical therapists.

68. In order to keep their jobs, nurse aides will need to follow institutional guidelines that may include all of the following EXCEPT
   a. reporting to work on time.
   b. following a dress code.
   c. reporting to the charge nurse.
   d. performing tasks without training.

69. Staff who are supervised by an RN are
   a. administration.
   b. physicians.
   c. assistive personnel.
   d. residents.

70. During a job interview, the nurse aide should never
   a. ask about possibilities for advancement.
   b. make negative comments about former supervisors.
   c. ask about job responsibilities.
   d. talk about his own strengths and weaknesses.

Answers

1. a. Clients in Fowler's position are lying with the head of the bed elevated to a 45- to 60-degree angle. This helps prevent aspiration after eating. Clients in the Sims position are lying on the side with the knee and thigh drawn upward toward the chest. Clients in a lateral position are lying flat on their side. Clients lying flat on their abdomen with their head turned to the side are lying in the prone position.

2. b. According to Dr. Kübler-Ross, there are five stages of death: denial, anger, bargaining, depression, and acceptance.

3. b. This position will provide balance and support for the client. The cane should be properly fitted. Choice **a** is incorrect; using a cane on the weak side will make it difficult for the client to support his weight while moving. Choice **c** is incorrect; the purpose of a cane is to provide support for persons who can walk but who are weak on one side. Choice **d** is incorrect; using a cane on the weak side will make it difficult for the client to support his weight while moving.

4. c. Increased exercise burns calories, thereby increasing the patient's appetite. Decreased activity can lead to decreased metabolism and thus lead to lack of appetite. Bad dentures can make eating painful and thus lead to lack of appetite. Decreased saliva can lead to dry mouth and thus a decreased appetite.

5. c. *Atrophy* is muscle wasting, which can be prevented by providing the patient with range-of-motion exercises. A *contracture* is the tightening of a muscle that makes it dysfunctional. An *orthotic* is an orthopedic appliance that is used to support, align, prevent, or correct deformities or to improve function of movable parts of the body. A *fracture* is a break in a bone.

6. b. The planning phase of the nursing process can be done only by the registered nurse. Nurse aides can participate in data collection, such as taking vital signs, and thus contribute to the assessment and evaluation process. They can make observations, such as reporting rashes, and thus contribute to the assessment process. Finally, nurse aides can carry out selected interventions, such as ambulating a client who has an order for ambulate with assistance.

7. c. Proper instructions for hand placement prevent nerve damage, which may cause paralysis to the arm. The armpits should not touch the top of the crutches, and the crutches should not rest upon the shoulders. Crutches are used to decrease weight bearing on the legs.

8. b. This is the maximum time a resident should be left in one position. Frequent turning promotes good circulation. Every hour is too frequent, unless there is a specific reason for this. Every three or four hours does not allow for proper circulation.

9. b. The main goal is independence, which should improve the client's sense of self. Choice **a** is incorrect; the ability to self-groom is, by itself, not a reason for early discharge. Choice **c** is incorrect; self-grooming may help with the acceptance of the disability, but it is not the main goal. Choice **d** is incorrect; self-grooming may help with the body image, but it is not the main goal.

10. a. While all of the answer choices are outcomes, the main goal of bladder training is to promote a regular pattern of continence.

11. d. Observing the patient helps prevent aspiration, while still allowing the client some independence in feeding himself. Choice **a** is incorrect; clients should not be asked to watch their roommates. Choice **b** is incorrect; feeding a client who can feed himself robs that client of his independence. Choice **c** is incorrect; the Heimlich maneuver is only used for airway obstruction.

12. b. This may be an indication of a serious condition and should be reported immediately. Burning and itching may be signs that something is wrong, and the problem may need immediate attention. Since the cause of the burning and tingling is not known at this point, rubbing and/or applying lotion or cornstarch may make it worse.

13. d. Inhaling the bacteria from the pillowcase can cause infection to the healthcare provider. Choice **a** is incorrect; holding the case under the chin will not cause a tear. Choice **b** is incorrect; the pillowcase may not drop. Choice **c** is incorrect; the chin will not dampen the pillowcase.

14. c. A clean dressing is nonsterile but promotes protection to the skin. An adhesive bandage is an example of a clean dressing. Wetting a dressing renders it nonsterile, but this is not the proper definition. A dry or a new dressing may or may not be sterile.

15. c. Use a clean portion of the cloth each time you wipe to prevent contamination. Choice **a** is incorrect; cleaning the eye from the outer corner to the inner corner risks spreading organisms across the eye. Choice **b** is incorrect; hydrogen peroxide can damage the eyes. Choice **d** is incorrect; if an eye has exudates, it should be cleaned last to avoid cross contamination.

16. d. In *modular nursing*, each member of the team carries out the same assigned task for all patients and residents. In *primary nursing*, one nurse is assigned several patients or residents, and other nurses or nurse aides work with these clients when the primary nurse is not on duty. In *patient-centered nursing*, care is designed to meet the patient's or resident's needs more efficiently. In *team nursing*, the same aide does not always perform the same task for every patient.

17. a. Pericare is performed to a body area contaminated by organisms, so nurse aides need to wear gloves to protect themselves and other clients. Gloves are not needed for routine bedmaking, washing a resident's hair, or feeding a patient.

18. d. The charge nurse needs to assess whether this is a normal behavior for this client or if something is wrong. No client should be left on a bedpan for a prolonged period of time. A waterproof underpad is used for clients who are incontinent. Extra rest will not help this situation.

19. d. All unusual behavior should be reported for evaluation. Choice **a** is incorrect; restraining a client without consent or a physician's order can be deemed wrongful imprisonment. Choice **b** is incorrect; this is a new behavior, and therefore it needs to be reported. Choice **c** is incorrect; it is not the nurse aide's role to discuss this with the family.

20. b. The Hoyer lift moves heavy or weak clients and those with mobility issues, while at the same time preventing healthcare worker injuries. The Hoyer lift can be used for clients who are very heavy, weak, or helpless. The use of a Hoyer lift can prevent back injuries to healthcare workers.

21. c. Active range-of-motion exercises require that the client do the exercises independently. Choice **a** is incorrect; moving joints to the point of pain may cause injury. Choice **b** is incorrect; the body should not be exposed to maintain the resident's privacy. Choice **d** is incorrect; proper body mechanics should always be used at their optimal level to prevent injury to the nurse aide.

22. a. A broad base of having the feet 12 inches apart will allow the center of gravity to assist in the transfer. Choice **b** is incorrect; the knees and hips should be bent to bring your center of gravity closer to your base of support. Choice **c** is incorrect; objects should be held close to the body to maintain the broad base of support. Choice **d** is incorrect; the feet should be about shoulder width apart, and the hands close to the body in relation to the object being held.

23. c. Changing the positions of the weights requires a physician's orders. Choice **a** is incorrect; clients in traction are usually on complete bedrest and thus need a bed bath. Choice **b** is incorrect; the skin should be monitored for color, especially at the area distal to the traction to assure there is adequate circulation. Choice **d** is incorrect; all possible distal pulses should be measured to check for adequate circulation. Measuring both sides of the body allows for comparison.

24. c. The pillow provides safety and prevents the client from striking her head on the bed. The pillow needs to be used to protect the head; it can be placed where the client desires after the move is completed.

25. d. Sitting the resident on the side of the bed allows the blood to drain to the lower extremities and prevents the client from fainting. The client is placed in a sitting position just prior to dangling. Still, a client who needs assistance to dangle may not be able to put on her own shoes. Although movement does increase circulation, dangling is not done to prevent decubiti.

26. a. The transfer belt provides a lift mechanism and prevents the client from falling while walking. Walking with a wheelchair a few steps behind a client will not help if the client falls. The Hoyer lift is used to transfer weak or heavy clients. Having a doctor or nurse ready for emergencies will do nothing to prevent them.

27. a. Cheerfulness need not be reported unless it is suddenly noted in a depressed client because then it may be a sign of suicidal thinking. Sudden paleness, excessive sweating, and increased respiratory rate are signs of potential problems that should be reported immediately.

28. b. Locking the brakes will prevent the chair from rolling and the client from falling. Unlocked brakes can cause the wheelchair to move when transferring the client, and this can result in the client falling. The Hoyer lift is only used for specific clients. Socks worn without shoes create a fall hazard.

29. d. Nurse aides do not report directly to physicians. The nurse aide should make sure the transfer is permissible for the client's condition, and he or she should know proper procedure before carrying out any client intervention. A transfer belt is used to assist with transfer, as well as standing and walking.

30. d. The *radial pulse* is located at the wrist and is most commonly used. The *carotid pulse* is located in the neck. The *apical pulse* is located in the chest, at the apex of the heart. The *femoral pulse* is located in the groin.

31. b. An *electrocardiogram* may also be called an EKG. It is the apparatus used in electrocardiography. EEG stands for *electroencephalogram*. It is the apparatus used to measure the electrical activity of the brain. *Electroconvulsive therapy* may also be called ECT. It is the common term for electroshock therapy. *Electromyogram* is also called EMG and is the term for a graph of the electric currents of muscle action.

32. a. The pulse indicates tachycardia and the BP is abnormally low. These vital signs need to be reported immediately. Choice **b** is incorrect; the temperature and pulse are within normal limits. The BP is elevated and should be reported, but it does not need to be reported immediately. Choices **c** and **d** are incorrect; these vital signs are within normal limits.

33. c. The drawsheet saves on bed changes and can be used as a lift sheet to move the client in bed. An underpad is a waterproof pad, usually disposable, that is used for incontinence. A spread is a decorative covering for a bed. A sheet covers the entire bed.

34. a. When the client is bedridden, the bed sheets need to be changed with the client in bed. This is called an occupied bedmaking procedure. When the client is ambulatory, the bed is made unoccupied, without the client lying on it. There is no circle procedure, and fitted sheets are not used by all facilities.

35. a. Constipation is a common post-op complication from the effects of anesthesia. Not taking in adequate fluids will increase the risk of this complication. Choice **b** is incorrect; blood clots are not formed by inadequate fluid intake post-op. They are formed when a client remains in one position for a prolonged period of time. Choice **c** is incorrect; infection is a common post-op complication, but it is not caused by inadequate fluid intake. It is caused by contamination with microorganisms. Choice **d** is incorrect; foot drop has many causes, but is not caused by inadequate fluids post-op.

36. b. Poor nail care can lead to infection in the diabetic client. Diabetic clients required licensed personnel to provide nail care. Cancer clients may have problems as a result of poor nail care if they are immunosuppressed, but they are not the most likely in this group. Stroke clients and developmentally disabled clients are not most likely to have problems as a result of poor nail care.

37. b. Encourage as much independence as possible. The nurse aide should do mouth care for a client only if the client cannot perform this herself. Clients should be encouraged, not told, to engage in self-care. The entire mouth needs oral care.

38. c. The trochanter roll prevents external hip rotation. A brace or splint would help keep the arm straight. Pillows would help keep a client on her side. The foot of the bed can be used to flex the legs.

39. a. A plate guard enables the client to better get the food off the plate with one hand. An arm brace is used to stabilize joints. A sling is used to immobilize the arm. A bib is used to protect the client's clothing during eating.

40. c. In many developmentally disabled clients, learning is slower than normal, but it still occurs and should be encouraged. Residents with developmental disabilities should be treated with respect like any other adult client. Developmental disability ranges from mild to severe. Most persons with developmental disability fall into the mild range and can master many of the skills needed for daily living. Persons with developmental disabilities are not necessarily suspicious of new people.

41. b. The diabetic patient needs time to accept the amputation and realize that it does not need to affect sexuality. Persons with disabilities still have sexuality, though losing her leg can affect her body image, which may affect her feelings of sexuality.

42. d. The Alzheimer's patient suffers from physical and mental decline. Alzheimer's disease is not typically associated with fever, chest pains, or difficulty breathing. Persons with Alzheimer's disease have difficulty with memory, beginning with recent memory.

43. d. Calm the patient down and allow her to voice her concerns in a constructive way. Sternly telling an upset client to quiet down may cause the client's distress to escalate. Offering to call her doctor will not solve her immediate needs. Shutting the client's door will disallow observation of the client, who may harm herself.

44. c. Lack of appetite may be caused by diseases, especially depression. Depression makes people lose interest in favored activities and is more likely to result in crying than laughing. Depressed clients often isolate themselves from others.

45. c. The nurse aide does not know when the patient may die. Allow her to die with dignity and respect her wishes. The client may not have time to wait for her family. The nurse aide should not give the client false hope.

46. a. Listening and empathy form the foundation for developing a sense of trust with clients, and trust is critical to their psychological well-being. Choice **b** is incorrect; everything may not be okay, and thus the nurse aide would be giving false assurance. Choice **c** is incorrect; maintaining confidentiality is important, but it is not used to assist the client with his psychological needs. Choice **d** is incorrect; the roommate is not responsible for the client.

47. b. The nurse aide should make every effort to respect the client's religious needs. The client is entitled to a healthy, balanced meal, and the facility will provide the client with a meatless lunch. She does not need to speak to a priest unless she desires to do so.

48. b. The nurse aide should respect the patient's sexuality rights and leave the room. The patient has a right to appropriately express his sexuality, and there is no need to report this to the nurse. Discussing it with another nurse aide violates the patient's confidentiality.

49. a. Including the client in her plan of care helps the client maintain dignity and feel a sense of independence. Serving her dinner first may single her out and make her feel different from the other clients. The client should be addressed by her title and surname, unless she requests to be called by her first name. Doing the client's care for her decreases her independence.

50. a. Gestures, facial expressions, and posture are all examples of body language. Writing is an expression of verbal communication. Sharing feelings is an example of verbal communication. Offering advice and opinions is an example of verbal communication.

51. a. Head nodding and smiling while someone is speaking to you demonstrates interest and says, "Tell me more." The nurse did not smile and nod continuously, and thus did not indicate agreement with everything the client said. The nurse aide is using nonverbal communication, which has nothing to do with lack of work.

52. c. *Making assumptions* can lead to conflict and confusion. *Reflection* is mirroring back what the client says. *Clarification* is verifying whether understanding is accurate. *Active listening* is being attentive to what the client is saying.

53. b. Confidentiality is important, and the charge nurse can explain that to visitors. Although the nurse aide is not allowed to talk to the friend about the client, choice **a** does not explain why this is true. Client information is confidential, and thus the nurse aide cannot disclose it to a client's friend. Telling the friend that you do not know what is wrong with the client is not truthful.

54. c. Asking the question will help determine if there are any underlying physical or psychological reasons why the client chooses not to bathe. The nurse aide should not force the client to take a bath. Stating that the client's roommate would not appreciate the smell is being verbally abusive. Asking the client if she thinks there is something wrong with taking a bath may make the client feel guilty.

55. a. *False imprisonment* is the act of restraining another person. Closing a client's door is not false imprisonment. Treating a client differently because of his religious beliefs is *discrimination*. Refusing to answer a call light that rings frequently may result in *negligence* if the client is injured because of the nurse aide's lack of action.

56. d. Inadequate care may result in client neglect and should be reported right away. Choice **a** is incorrect; in the time it takes to make a list, the other nurse aide is providing inadequate care to clients. Choice **b** is incorrect; staff members other than the charge nurse cannot act on a situation where a nurse aide is not providing adequate care. Choice **c** is incorrect; completing the care himself will not stop the other nurse aide's negative behavior.

57. b. *Objective* information is what the nurse sees, hears, smells, and feels. *Subjective* observation comes from what the client tells you. *Primary* observation relates to what should be considered first. *Secondary* observation relates to what is considered after primary observation.

58. b. Since the resident is a former leader, the resident may feel better if feeling useful and involved. Reading industrial magazines and watching business-oriented movies may be of interest to the resident, but this will not help to maintain his dignity. Relaxing and playing bingo may relieve his stress, but this will not help maintain his dignity, either.

59. d. The nurse will evaluate the client's condition and the daughter's abilities, then decide what the daughter can safely do for her mother. Choice **a** is incorrect; the daughter may not know how to do the care correctly and may cause injury to her mother. Choice **b** is incorrect; family members can perform care for their loved ones. Choice **c** is incorrect; the daughter should be able to do all the care she is capable of doing and the nurse agrees to let her do.

60. b. Terminally ill clients have physical and psychological needs that need to be met. The client may not want to be alone during the last stage of a terminal illness, and the client may not want to be cared for by family or friends. Terminally ill clients should have choices about their care.

61. b. Personal clothing enhances the client's sense of well-being. While allowing personal clothing may decrease clothing costs somewhat, this is not the reason why clients are allowed to wear their own clothing. Personal clothing may actually make it more difficult to dress clients than hospital gowns. Personal clothing does not necessarily enhance infection control.

62. a. Always knock on a closed door and wait for a response to ensure client privacy. Choice **b** is incorrect; the nurse aide should not assume anything, as the client may be in distress behind the closed door. Choice **c** is incorrect; immediately opening the door and walking right in violates the client's privacy. Choice **d** is incorrect; the nurse aide should first wait for the client to respond.

63. d. Restraints should be used only when a resident's safety is involved. A restraint must be ordered by a physician. Using a restraint for staff convenience can be deemed false imprisonment and abuse.

64. c. As long as it is a safe choice, allow the client to make personal choices. The client has a right to choose her own clothing. Telling the client she will look uncoordinated may insult the client. Selecting another outfit for the client robs the client of her independence.

65. b. *Malpractice* is the failure to give service for which one is trained. *Discrimination* is a prejudiced outlook or behavior. *Defamation* is harming a person's reputation by words that you say (slander) or write (libel) intentionally. *False imprisonment* is the act of restraining another person.

66. b. As long as the client is safe, provide privacy while the client is on the commode. Leaving the curtain open while a client uses the commode deprives the client of privacy. Making the client's bed while the client is on the commode distracts the nurse aide from the client, who may fall. The client is allowed to use the commode as needed.

67. c. The healthcare team is the group of caregivers involved in providing care to patients. Nurse aides, physicians, and physical therapists are all members of the healthcare team.

68. d. Nurse aides should not perform tasks for which they have not been adequately trained. Reporting to work on time, following a dress code, and reporting to the charge nurse are expected roles of the nurse aide.

69. c. LPNs and CNAs are assistive personnel. The RN is responsible for delegating assignments to qualified staff. RNs report to the administration and follow physician orders. Residents report to attending physicians.

70. b. Making negative comments about another person during a job interview will only cast a negative image upon the interviewee. Keep the interview positive. It is appropriate and encouraged for nurse aides to ask about possible advancement. Nurse aides should ask about their job responsibilities so that they may accomplish them and should talk about their own strengths and weaknesses as a way of self-improvement.

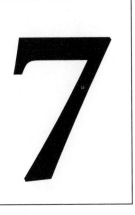

NURSING ASSISTANT/NURSE AIDE PRACTICE EXAM 5

CHAPTER SUMMARY

This is the fifth and final nursing assistant exam. By the time you finish this exam, you should be prepared for the real thing.

This is the last sample National Nurse Aide Assesment Program (NNAAP) written exam in this book. For this last test, pull together all the tips you have been practicing since the first test. Give yourself the time and the space to work, perhaps in an unfamiliar location such as a library, since you won't be taking the real test in your living room. In addition, draw on what you have learned from reading the answer explanations. Remember the types of questions that you struggled with in the past, and when you are unsure, try to consider how those answers were explained.

When you are done, check your answers and refer to the Appendix (page 159) to find out on which sections you may need a final review. Most of all, relax. You have worked hard and have every right to be confident—good luck!

Practice Exam 5

1.	ⓐ	ⓑ	ⓒ	ⓓ	26.	ⓐ	ⓑ	ⓒ	ⓓ	51.	ⓐ	ⓑ	ⓒ	ⓓ
2.	ⓐ	ⓑ	ⓒ	ⓓ	27.	ⓐ	ⓑ	ⓒ	ⓓ	52.	ⓐ	ⓑ	ⓒ	ⓓ
3.	ⓐ	ⓑ	ⓒ	ⓓ	28.	ⓐ	ⓑ	ⓒ	ⓓ	53.	ⓐ	ⓑ	ⓒ	ⓓ
4.	ⓐ	ⓑ	ⓒ	ⓓ	29.	ⓐ	ⓑ	ⓒ	ⓓ	54.	ⓐ	ⓑ	ⓒ	ⓓ
5.	ⓐ	ⓑ	ⓒ	ⓓ	30.	ⓐ	ⓑ	ⓒ	ⓓ	55.	ⓐ	ⓑ	ⓒ	ⓓ
6.	ⓐ	ⓑ	ⓒ	ⓓ	31.	ⓐ	ⓑ	ⓒ	ⓓ	56.	ⓐ	ⓑ	ⓒ	ⓓ
7.	ⓐ	ⓑ	ⓒ	ⓓ	32.	ⓐ	ⓑ	ⓒ	ⓓ	57.	ⓐ	ⓑ	ⓒ	ⓓ
8.	ⓐ	ⓑ	ⓒ	ⓓ	33.	ⓐ	ⓑ	ⓒ	ⓓ	58.	ⓐ	ⓑ	ⓒ	ⓓ
9.	ⓐ	ⓑ	ⓒ	ⓓ	34.	ⓐ	ⓑ	ⓒ	ⓓ	59.	ⓐ	ⓑ	ⓒ	ⓓ
10.	ⓐ	ⓑ	ⓒ	ⓓ	35.	ⓐ	ⓑ	ⓒ	ⓓ	60.	ⓐ	ⓑ	ⓒ	ⓓ
11.	ⓐ	ⓑ	ⓒ	ⓓ	36.	ⓐ	ⓑ	ⓒ	ⓓ	61.	ⓐ	ⓑ	ⓒ	ⓓ
12.	ⓐ	ⓑ	ⓒ	ⓓ	37.	ⓐ	ⓑ	ⓒ	ⓓ	62.	ⓐ	ⓑ	ⓒ	ⓓ
13.	ⓐ	ⓑ	ⓒ	ⓓ	38.	ⓐ	ⓑ	ⓒ	ⓓ	63.	ⓐ	ⓑ	ⓒ	ⓓ
14.	ⓐ	ⓑ	ⓒ	ⓓ	39.	ⓐ	ⓑ	ⓒ	ⓓ	64.	ⓐ	ⓑ	ⓒ	ⓓ
15.	ⓐ	ⓑ	ⓒ	ⓓ	40.	ⓐ	ⓑ	ⓒ	ⓓ	65.	ⓐ	ⓑ	ⓒ	ⓓ
16.	ⓐ	ⓑ	ⓒ	ⓓ	41.	ⓐ	ⓑ	ⓒ	ⓓ	66.	ⓐ	ⓑ	ⓒ	ⓓ
17.	ⓐ	ⓑ	ⓒ	ⓓ	42.	ⓐ	ⓑ	ⓒ	ⓓ	67.	ⓐ	ⓑ	ⓒ	ⓓ
18.	ⓐ	ⓑ	ⓒ	ⓓ	43.	ⓐ	ⓑ	ⓒ	ⓓ	68.	ⓐ	ⓑ	ⓒ	ⓓ
19.	ⓐ	ⓑ	ⓒ	ⓓ	44.	ⓐ	ⓑ	ⓒ	ⓓ	69.	ⓐ	ⓑ	ⓒ	ⓓ
20.	ⓐ	ⓑ	ⓒ	ⓓ	45.	ⓐ	ⓑ	ⓒ	ⓓ	70.	ⓐ	ⓑ	ⓒ	ⓓ
21.	ⓐ	ⓑ	ⓒ	ⓓ	46.	ⓐ	ⓑ	ⓒ	ⓓ					
22.	ⓐ	ⓑ	ⓒ	ⓓ	47.	ⓐ	ⓑ	ⓒ	ⓓ					
23.	ⓐ	ⓑ	ⓒ	ⓓ	48.	ⓐ	ⓑ	ⓒ	ⓓ					
24.	ⓐ	ⓑ	ⓒ	ⓓ	49.	ⓐ	ⓑ	ⓒ	ⓓ					
25.	ⓐ	ⓑ	ⓒ	ⓓ	50.	ⓐ	ⓑ	ⓒ	ⓓ					

Practice Exam 5

1. It is important to practice standard precautions when
  a. dressing a patient.
  b. feeding a patient.
  c. providing oral hygiene.
  d. ambulating a patient.

2. What position should a patient be in to receive an enema?
  a. supine
  b. Fowler's
  c. prone
  d. left Sim's

3. Which of the following lists only items that would be included in fluid intake?
  a. milk, ham sandwich, ice cream bar
  b. water, mashed potatoes, gelatin
  c. milk, custard, soup
  d. orange juice, soft-boiled egg, toast

4. The nurse aide must use a stethoscope to determine the
  a. apical pulse rate.
  b. carotid pulse rate.
  c. popliteal pulse rate.
  d. brachial pulse rate.

5. Another name for urination is
  a. defecation.
  b. voiding.
  c. enuresis.
  d. flatus.

6. A client complains of a sore spot in her calf. The nurse aide should
  a. massage her legs with lotion.
  b. ask the nurse to check the client immediately.
  c. have the client walk to relieve the cramp.
  d. assess the soreness every hour for a few hours.

7. An example of possible contamination through direct contact is
  a. cleaning a bedpan.
  b. touching used linens.
  c. being sneezed on.
  d. using a doorknob.

8. A nurse aide finds smoke and flames coming from a resident's room. The nurse aide should first
  a. attempt to get the resident out of the room and close the door.
  b. get the fire extinguisher and put out the fire.
  c. take away the resident's cigarettes.
  d. pull the fire alarm.

9. To place a client in good alignment, the nurse aide should
  a. keep the client's joints well lubricated.
  b. keep the client as straight as possible.
  c. keep the bed linens wrinkle free.
  d. ambulate the client at least twice a day.

10. When dressing a client with left-sided weakness, it is important for the nurse aide to begin dressing him
  a. on the right side.
  b. on the left side.
  c. when he is lying flat in bed.
  d. as he lies on either side.

11. Which of the following conditions needs to be reported immediately to the charge nurse?
    a. rash that appears suddenly
    b. warm, dry, pink skin
    c. tough skin on the feet
    d. scarred skin

12. A nurse aide is making rounds at 1:00 A.M. She finds a patient lighting a cigarette. Assuming smoking is allowed in the facility, what should she do?
    a. Scold him and tell him never to smoke unsupervised again.
    b. Remain with the patient until he finishes smoking.
    c. Tell another coworker.
    d. Call the charge nurse to supervise.

13. A client with a broken hip needs an enema. The best bedpan to use would be a
    a. fracture pan.
    b. plastic pan.
    c. pediatric pan.
    d. metal pan.

14. Which of the following is true about visually challenged clients?
    a. They prefer to eat alone.
    b. They use a "clock" system to find their food.
    c. They prefer to be fed.
    d. They need liquid diets.

15. Before ambulating a client who has a Foley catheter, the nurse aide should first
    a. clamp off the catheter and disconnect it.
    b. let the bag dangle between the client's legs.
    c. carry the bag below bladder level.
    d. hide the bag in a pillow case.

16. A resident is walking back and forth in the hall. The nurse aide should
    a. restrain the resident.
    b. walk with the resident.
    c. place the resident in a locked room.
    d. continue to observe the client.

17. When transferring a client, the client becomes weak and begins to fall. The nurse aide's first action is to
    a. hold the transfer belt and lean against the wall.
    b. call for help.
    c. grasp the transfer belt and lower the client to the floor.
    d. hold the client tightly to prevent falling.

18. The best way to measure accurate daily weights is to
    a. weigh the client without clothing.
    b. weigh the client fully clothed.
    c. weigh the client at the same time each day.
    d. weigh the client after breakfast.

19. A client is sitting in her room with a doll in her arms, stating, "My baby is sick." What should the nurse aide do?
    a. Tell her not to worry because the baby will be fine.
    b. Tell her that the aide will call the baby's doctor.
    c. Ask her if she is upset with her doll.
    d. Tell her the baby is not real.

20. Padded side rails are used to
    a. keep the client in bed.
    b. protect the client from injury.
    c. provide additional warmth.
    d. remind the client of home.

21. A nurse aide is recording the output of a resident who has a Foley catheter. She sees that the urine bag is empty. What should she do first?
    a. Irrigate the catheter.
    b. Check for kinks in the tube.
    c. Replace the drainage bag.
    d. Replace the catheter.

22. In the middle of lunch, a client stands up, clutching her neck and unable to speak. The nurse aide should first
    a. call for help.
    b. offer her a drink of water.
    c. hit her on the back.
    d. perform the Heimlich maneuver.

23. A client has not had a bowel movement in five days. He may also complain of
    a. nausea.
    b. headache.
    c. leg cramps.
    d. chest pain.

24. A client who is weak and unsteady needs to urinate. The nurse aide can safely leave him alone to use a
    a. commode.
    b. toilet.
    c. bedpan.
    d. urinal.

25. For a client who is classified as wound-and-skin isolation, the soiled linen should be
    a. placed in the linen hamper.
    b. discarded.
    c. bagged before removing from the room.
    d. taken directly to the laundry.

26. If a resident begins to choke while being fed and is unable to speak, the nurse aide should call for help and begin doing
    a. back blows.
    b. mouth-to-mouth ventilations.
    c. a finger sweep.
    d. abdominal thrusts.

27. When making a bed, the nurse aide should place the soiled linen
    a. on the bedside table.
    b. on the floor.
    c. in a laundry bag.
    d. in a red plastic bag.

28. The ABCs of emergency care stand for
    a. airway, breathing, circulation.
    b. action before calling.
    c. airway before circulation.
    d. action, benefits, contact.

29. When forcing fluids, the nurse aide should offer
    a. clear fluids only.
    b. at least 5,000 cc of fluid per shift.
    c. fluids every hour.
    d. high-calorie fluids.

30. When caring for a hearing-impaired client, the nursing assistant should do all of the following EXCEPT
    a. stand or sit facing the client.
    b. speak clearly and slowly.
    c. raise your voice.
    d. use simple words and sentences.

31. Security for a client's dentures includes
    a. keeping them in a tissue in a dresser drawer.
    b. placing them in a labeled denture cup.
    c. insisting the client wear the dentures.
    d. placing an identifying mark on the dentures.

32. While caring for a client, a nurse aide accidentally gets blood in her eyes. The nurse aide should first
   a. rinse them out with clear water.
   b. call 911.
   c. report the incident to the charge nurse.
   d. document it.

33. A client drinks four ounces of juice. The nurse aide would document this as
   a. 4 ounces.
   b. four ounces.
   c. one cup.
   d. 120 cc.

34. When using client restraints, the nurse aide should
   a. observe for skin irritation.
   b. disallow the client to drink.
   c. release the restraints every four hours.
   d. leave the client alone to rest.

35. Which of the following vital signs should be reported immediately?
   a. T–98.6, P–70, R–14, BP–120/60
   b. T–95.4, P–40, R–10, BP–80/40
   c. T–98.8 "R," P–60, R–20, BP–132/70
   d. T–97.6 "ax," P–78, R–16, BP–110/60

36. Examples of client abuse include all of the following EXCEPT
   a. forcing a client's fingers off the side rails.
   b. deliberately leaving the call bell out of reach.
   c. turning the lights out against the client's wishes.
   d. using gloves when providing pericare.

37. When bathing a client, the nurse aide recognizes which of the following as the first sign of a pressure ulcer?
   a. redness
   b. swelling
   c. numbness
   d. pain

38. Nurse aides should wash their hands in all of the following situations EXCEPT
   a. before going to the bathroom.
   b. after each client contact.
   c. before eating.
   d. after changing dressings.

39. While bathing a resident, the nursing assistant notices a rash on the resident's legs. The nursing assistant should
   a. ignore it if the resident does not complain.
   b. wash it to see if it disappears.
   c. rub it with alcohol to dry it out.
   d. notify the charge nurse of the rash.

40. The nursing assistant should tell clients
   a. how to dress.
   b. how to call for help.
   c. that things will get better.
   d. that there is nothing to worry about.

41. A client begins to have a seizure while the nurse aide is bathing him. The nurse aide should
   a. hold him down to prevent him from falling.
   b. put a tongue depressor in his mouth.
   c. protect him from injuring himself.
   d. run out of the room and get help.

42. Sputum is best collected
   a. just before bedtime.
   b. in the afternoon.
   c. upon awakening in the morning.
   d. anytime.

43. To change direction, a nurse aide should
   a. turn her whole body by moving her feet.
   b. twist from the waist.
   c. move her body in sections.
   d. move her body very slowly.

44. When repositioning a heavy client, the nurse aide should
   a. attempt to move the client alone.
   b. let the family move the client.
   c. get another aide to help.
   d. move the client later.

45. To help a client into a wheelchair, the nurse aide should position the chair
   a. at the side of the bed, facing the head of the bed.
   b. at the foot of the bed.
   c. at the head of the bed.
   d. at the side of the bed, facing the foot of the bed.

46. Transferring a client from a bed to a stretcher requires that the nurse aide use
   a. proper body mechanics.
   b. a Hoyer lift.
   c. a minimum of three coworkers.
   d. a mobility mattress.

47. Which statement about dressing residents is correct?
   a. Dressing is a waste of time for a handicapped resident.
   b. Residents are used to dressing in front of others.
   c. Residents care about what they wear.
   d. Residents like the nurse aide to dress them.

48. Which of the following is an example of a client's delusion?
   a. seeing demons
   b. feeling imaginary bugs crawl on his arms
   c. thinking that the CIA is secretly watching him
   d. hearing voices demand that he escape from the facility

49. Reality orientation techniques include all of the following EXCEPT
   a. labeling items in the client's room.
   b. putting up calendars and clocks.
   c. using familiar items in the client's room.
   d. reminding a client that his spouse is deceased.

50. A young resident with muscular dystrophy talks about wanting a boyfriend. This feeling is best described as
   a. normal.
   b. hopeless.
   c. unrealistic.
   d. confused.

51. A nurse aide walks in on a client masturbating in his bathroom. The nurse aide should
   a. insist that the client stop.
   b. ask the client why he is engaging in this behavior.
   c. report it to the charge nurse.
   d. allow the client privacy.

52. When providing postmortem care, the nurse aide must
   a. ensure that a family member is present.
   b. have a coworker assist her.
   c. wear gloves.
   d. contact the funeral director for instructions.

53. Which statement about bathing unconscious clients is correct?
- **a.** Unconscious clients may be able to hear you speaking to them during the bath.
- **b.** Unconscious clients can turn in bed when asked.
- **c.** Unconscious clients do not need to be observed for decubiti.
- **d.** Unconscious clients have very moist skin.

54. A client wants to know what is wrong with his roommate. The nurse aide's best response is
- **a.** "It is really nothing for you to worry about."
- **b.** "I'll check with his doctor for you."
- **c.** "Sorry, I can't share that information with you."
- **d.** "You can call his doctor and ask yourself."

55. The care plan includes all of the following EXCEPT
- **a.** the nursing diagnosis.
- **b.** short- and long-term goals.
- **c.** cost of the hospital stay.
- **d.** scheduled appointments for the resident.

56. A ten-month-old baby cries and pulls at his left ear. The nurse aide should
- **a.** give the baby ear drops.
- **b.** put a warm cloth on the baby's ear.
- **c.** give the baby a bottle.
- **d.** report it to the charge nurse.

57. A client is hard of hearing and repeatedly turns her call light on. The nurse aide should
- **a.** take time to listen to her to determine her needs.
- **b.** talk loudly to her since she is hard of hearing.
- **c.** unplug the call light.
- **d.** tell the supervisor that the client is uncooperative.

58. When giving a client a bath, the nurse aide should do all of the following EXCEPT
- **a.** ensure the client's privacy.
- **b.** check the water temperature.
- **c.** gather all supplies before starting.
- **d.** perform a mental status exam.

59. A client who is eating poorly should be offered
- **a.** vitamin pills.
- **b.** tube feeding.
- **c.** clear broth.
- **d.** dietary supplements.

60. What are the signs of death?
- **a.** convulsions
- **b.** loss of consciousness
- **c.** no respirations, pulse, or blood pressure
- **d.** no response when you call the patient

61. On Good Friday, a Catholic client is served chicken and requests a meatless meal. The nurse aide should
- **a.** offer to get another meal within the client's diet.
- **b.** call the client's priest for a dispensation.
- **c.** tell the client that it is all right since she is in the hospital.
- **d.** tell her the aide will check with the dietician for the next day's meal.

62. A client is observing the Islamic holy month of Ramadan by fasting from sunup to sundown. The most appropriate action for the nurse aide would be to
- **a.** contact the dietician for a special tray.
- **b.** report this to the charge nurse.
- **c.** find out when the client may eat and drink.
- **d.** inform the client that she must eat her prescribed diet.

63. An ECF resident tells the nurse aide something about her family in confidence. The nurse aide
a. can tell any staff member.
b. ethically cannot tell anyone else.
c. can tell the charge nurse only.
d. can tell anyone who does not know the resident.

64. A nurse aide observes a client falling in the hallway. It is important that the nurse aide report
a. what the nurse aide thinks happened.
b. exactly what the nurse aide observed.
c. nothing, if this is not the nurse aide's client.
d. what may have happened that day.

65. A client's daughter offers the nurse aide $50 to thank her for caring for the client. The nurse aide should
a. accept it to be polite.
b. politely refuse it.
c. use the money for the client.
d. report this to the charge nurse.

66. An elderly resident recently cared for her husband until he died. The nurse aide recognizes that this client needs to
a. keep busy to keep her mind off her husband.
b. have adequate time alone to grieve for her husband.
c. meet other men to find a new partner.
d. keep from crying to avoid getting more upset.

67. A resident refuses to go to physical therapy one morning. The nurse aide reports this to the charge nurse, who discusses this with the resident. The resident states that she will go to physical therapy the next day. The nurse aide understands that the resident
a. has the right to refuse treatment.
b. should not be given choices in his therapy.
c. does not have the right to refuse therapy.
d. can refuse therapy only with the doctor's permission.

68. A person admitted to a hospital or extended-care facility can be expected to be treated according to the
a. State Hospital Association.
b. Caregiver's Bill of Rights.
c. Patient's Bill of Rights.
d. Physician's Association.

69. The nurse aide is told to bring a client by wheelchair to the X-Ray Department and covers the client with a robe, blanket, and slippers. The nurse aide has maintained the client's
a. right to confidentiality.
b. right to privacy.
c. right to nursing care plans.
d. right to refuse.

70. Nurse aides need to identify themselves with their names and title of CNA before giving any care to clients. This is an example of the patient's right to
a. considerate and respectful care.
b. privacy.
c. identification of healthcare workers.
d. be informed of hospital policies.

Answers

1. c. When coming in contact with oral mucosa, it is possible to come in contact with blood-borne pathogens. Infection control must be implemented. Standard precautions are not needed when dressing or feeding a patient, unless the nurse aide will be exposed to bodily fluids. Standard precautions are not needed when ambulating a patient.

2. d. Left Sims allows for better irrigation of the colon. In the supine position, the patient is lying on his back, which does not allow for adequate irrigation of the colon. In the Fowler's position, the head of the bed is elevated to between 45 and 60 degrees, which does not allow for adequate irrigation of the colon. In the prone position the patient is lying on her abdomen, which does not allow for adequate irrigation of the colon.

3. c. Milk, custard, and soup are all fluids. A ham sandwich, mashed potatoes, a soft-boiled egg, and toast are not fluids.

4. a. The apical pulse rate can only be heard with a stethoscope. A stethoscope is used to listen for bruits in the carotid artery, but is not routinely used to assess the carotid pulse rate. Finger palpation is used to assess the popliteal pulse rate and the brachial pulse rate.

5. b. *Voiding* means urinating. *Defecating* means stooling. *Enuresis* means wetting the bed, as does incontinence. *Flatus* means expelling gas.

6. b. The nurse aide should report client complaints as soon as possible, and a sore calf may be a sign of a thrombus (blood clot), which can have serious complications. Choice **a** is incorrect; the sore spot may be a clot and massaging the area can dislodge the clot and cause it to travel to the lungs or other organ, which may prove fatal. Choice **c** is incorrect; walking to relieve the pain may also dislodge the clot. Choice **d** is incorrect; waiting to assess the clot runs the risk of the clot dislodging and traveling to an organ.

7. c. Sneezing is an example of direct contact, with potential contamination from secretions that come directly from the client. Contamination through cleaning a bedpan, touching used linens, and using a doorknob are examples of indirect contact.

8. a. Always try to rescue the victim first if possible, then call the fire department. Choice **b** is incorrect; the nurse aide should try to rescue the victim and call the fire department before trying to extinguish the fire. Choice **c** is incorrect; the nurse aide cannot take away a resident's personal belongings. Choice **d** is incorrect; attempt to rescue the victim before pulling the fire alarm.

9. b. Proper body alignment means that the client is kept as straight as possible to promote circulation and prevent contractures. Keeping joints well lubricated helps to prevent contractures, but it does not place a client in good alignment. Keeping the bed wrinkle free helps to prevent pressure sores, but it does not place a client in good alignment. Ambulating the client twice a day can help prevent many problems, but it does not place a client in good alignment.

10. b. When a client has one-sided weakness, it is important to begin dressing the client on the affected side to ease dressing and minimize pain. Choice **a** is incorrect; beginning with the unaffected side makes it more difficult to dress the affected side. Choice **c** is incorrect; it is more difficult to dress the client in a lying position. Choice **d** is incorrect; it is more difficult to dress the client when he is lying on either side.

11. a. A suddenly appearing rash is an acute change and should be reported immediately. Warm, dry, pink skin is a normal finding, and thus does not require immediate reporting. Tough skin on the feet develops over a period of time. It does not warrant immediate reporting, but does require reporting, especially if the client is diabetic. Scarred skin represents an old injury or surgery and thus does not require immediate reporting.

12. b. Most facilities are smoke free; however, depending on the situation, smoking may be permitted. It is the responsibility of the nurse aide to remain with the patient and put the cigarette out in the proper receptacle. Choice **a** is incorrect; scolding a patient is inappropriate. Choice **c** is incorrect; another coworker is not needed to manage this situation. Choice **d** is incorrect; the nurse aide should remain with the client until he finishes smoking and then report the smoking to the charge nurse.

13. a. Choose a fracture pan so that the client will have a minimal distance to lift his hips. A plastic or metal pan is too high for the client to lift his hips. A pediatric bedpan is too small for the client to use.

14. b. Visually impaired clients can feed themselves if they can visualize their food on a plate, and the "clock" system helps them do this. Choice **a** is incorrect; visually challenged clients enjoy the same socialization as clients who are not visually challenged. Choice **c** is incorrect; most clients prefer to be as independent as possible. Choice **d** is incorrect; there is no reason for visually impaired clients to need a liquid diet simply because of their visual impairment.

15. c. A nurse aide cannot disconnect the bag without an order, but he or she still must ensure that the bag remains below the bladder level. The inside of the catheter and tubing are sterile, and thus it is safer to not disconnect the tubing. Allowing the bag to dangle can cause the catheter to dislodge from the client. The bag should be hidden under the client's robe once the client is standing.

16. d. The nurse aide should continue to observe the client. This type of repetitive behavior cannot cause harm. Restraints cannot be applied without consent or a physician's order. The client may not want anyone to walk with him. Placing the client in a locked room can be deemed wrongful imprisonment.

17. c. Grasp the transfer belt and lower the resident to the floor along your bent leg. The nurse aide should not lean the client against the wall, and the nurse aide should call for help after lowering the client to the floor. Holding a falling client may result in injury to both the client and the nurse aide.

18. c. Weighing the client at the same time each day provides the best assessment of weight loss or gain. Weighing the client without any clothing deprives the client of privacy and dignity, and weighing the client fully clothed results in an inaccurately higher weight because of the weight of the clothes. Clients should be weighed before breakfast.

19. c. Asking the resident if she's upset with her doll can make her aware that it is not real, and help her cope with what is bothering her. Telling her not to worry will not allow the nurse aide to find out what is bothering the client, and it will reinforce her belief that the doll is real. Stating that you will call the baby's doctor will reinforce her belief that the doll is real. Confronting her directly that the baby is not real can be traumatic.

20. b. Padded side rails prevent clients, especially those who are confused, from injuring themselves on the bed rails. Side rails are used to prevent falls. Padded bed rails do not result in increased body warmth, and padded railing will not remind someone of home.

21. b. The nurse aide should always make sure there are no kinks that could prevent the flow of urine. Choice **a** is incorrect; the nurse aide is not responsible for irrigating catheters. Choice **c** is incorrect; replacing the drainage bag opens the system and increases the risk of infection. Choice **d** is incorrect; nurse aides do not replace catheters.

22. d. Hands at the throat are a universal sign of choking. The nurse aide should perform the Heimlich maneuver and call for help. Never leave the patient unattended. The nurse aide should call for help after performing the Heimlich maneuver. The client is choking and cannot drink water, and hitting her on the back will not dislodge the foreign body.

23. a. Abdominal fullness can cause nausea. Not having a bowel movement in five days should not result in chest pain, a headache, or leg cramps.

24. c. Keep the client in bed to prevent a fall, but allow privacy while voiding. A weak and unsteady client may fall off of the commode or may fall en route to the bathroom. A weak client may also not be able to hold a urinal.

25. a. Wound-and-skin isolation means high likelihood of linen contamination, but according to Standard Precautions, all linen is considered potentially infective. Choice **b** is incorrect; soiled linen can be properly cleaned and does not need to be discarded. Choice **c** is incorrect; all linen is considered potentially infective and thus it does not require separate bagging. Choice **d** is incorrect; it is not the nurse aide's role to deliver soiled linen directly to the laundry.

26. d. Abdominal thrusts are always the first step for airway obstructions. Back blows are not used for adults. Mouth-to-mouth ventilations are not used in a conscious patient, and mouth-to-mouth ventilations will not work if the airway is obstructed. A finger sweep is conducted in an unconscious person if the object is visible.

27. c. Soiled linen should be directly placed in laundry bags to prevent contamination. Placing soiled linen on the bedside table can cause the table to become contaminated with microorganisms from the soiled linen, and soiled linen should not be placed on the floor, as it can cause a fall hazard. All linen is considered contaminated, thus red bagging is unnecessary.

28. a. ABC stands for airway (open airway), breathing (mouth to mouth), and circulation (chest compressions). Choice **b** is incorrect; the American Heart Association recommends first activating the emergency response system. Choice **c** is incorrect; airway does come before circulation, but that is not exactly what ABC stands for. Choice **d** is incorrect; ABC does not stand for action, benefits, contact.

29. c. Offer fluids every hour to better ensure the client is taking an adequate amount. Choice **a** is incorrect; unless otherwise stated, an order of forced fluids does not mean restriction to clear fluids. Choice **b** is incorrect; 5,000 cc of fluid per shift is too much fluid. Choice **d** is incorrect; high-calorie fluids may be too filling and may result in decreased fluid intake.

30. c. Speaking slowly and clearly will help a hearing-impaired client to understand. Simple words and sentences will also help. Facing the client allows the client to hear more clearly, and to read the nurse's lips, if possible.

31. b. Every resident with dentures must have a labeled denture cup to ensure security of the costly dentures. Choice **a** is incorrect; keeping dentures in a tissue in the drawer risks their breakage. Dentures are expensive. Choice **c** is incorrect; the nurse aide should not insist the client wear his dentures. Choice **d** is incorrect; nothing should be written directly on the dentures.

32. a. The nurse aide should rinse her eyes with water immediately, then report to the nurse for safety. It is not necessary to call 911 for a health emergency when inside a healthcare agency. The incident should be documented after the client's eyes are rinsed with water.

33. d. Fluid intake is documented in the metric system, and four ounces equals 120 cc. Ounces belong to the customary system. One cup is approximately 240 cc.

34. a. Restraints can cause skin irritations, so all restrained body parts must be observed for irritations. Choice **b** is incorrect; clients need fluids so that they do not dehydrate. Choice **c** is incorrect; restraints are removed every two hours. Choice **d** is incorrect; clients in restraints should be checked every 15 minutes to assure that feeling and blood flow are normal in each extremity, and that the client is not experiencing any difficulty.

35. b. The patient's vital signs are very low. Choice **a** is incorrect; these vital signs are within normal limits. Choice **c** is incorrect; the temperature, pulse, and respirations are normal. The systolic blood pressure is elevated and should be reported, but does not need to be reported immediately. Choice **d** is incorrect; these vital signs are within normal limits.

36. d. Using gloves for pericare is standard precaution, not client abuse. Choice **a** is incorrect; forcing a client's fingers off the side rails is physical abuse. Choice **b** is incorrect; deliberately leaving the call bell out of reach is abusive. Choice **c** is incorrect; turning the lights out against the client's wishes is psychological abuse.

37. a. Redness is usually the first sign of a pressure ulcer (Stage 1). Swelling is not a common finding in pressure ulcers. Pressure ulcers can occur in areas of numbness, and numbness may occur in the late stages if nerves are damaged. Pain may be noted during Stage 1, but redness is the first sign.

38. a. Wash your hands after going to the bathroom. The nurse aide should wash her hands after client contact as part of Standard Precautions. The nurse aide should wash her hands before eating to avoid contaminating her food. The nurse aide should wash her hands after changing dressings to prevent cross contamination.

39. d. All changes must be reported to the charge nurse. A rash can be a sign of a serious problem, even if it does not bother the client. It will not disappear with washing, and washing may irritate it. Alcohol can be irritating and a nurse aide should not apply alcohol without being instructed to do so.

40. b. The call bell system should be explained to the resident to keep a line of communication open. Clients can choose how to dress, and it is not the nurse aide's role to discuss illness progress with clients. Telling clients there is nothing to worry about decreases the likelihood that they will openly discuss their feelings.

41. c. Do not restrain the patient. Move all furniture and equipment away to protect him from injury. The client should be gently helped to the floor to prevent him from falling. Putting a tongue depressor in the client's mouth is an old practice that is no longer used. Call for help after you assure the client is safe, but do not leave the client alone.

42. c. It is best to collect sputum in the morning. This way, there are more bacteria in the specimen. Clients tend to have less sputum at the end of the day, and sputum tends to decrease throughout the day.

43. a. Moving the whole body prevents twisting the back muscles and an injury. Twisting from the waist can cause back strain. Moving your body in sections can cause injury. Moving very slowly is not helpful.

44. c. To prevent self-injury, the nurse aide should get another aide to assist in moving the client. Choice **a** is incorrect; the nurse aide may injure herself if she attempts to move a heavy client alone. Choice **b** is incorrect; the family is not responsible for moving the client. Choice **d** is incorrect; moving the client later does not change the dynamics of proper body mechanics.

45. d. Proximity of the bed to the chair will allow easier client transfer and the client will be facing the front of the room. The wheelchair should be placed at the side of the bed, but facing it toward the head of the bed will make transfer more difficult. Placing the wheelchair at the foot of the bed makes the transfer more difficult, because it is too far from the client. Placing the wheelchair at the head of the bed makes the transfer more difficult because it is too far from the client.

46. a. Body mechanics promote good musculoskeletal alignment. Choice **b** is incorrect; a Hoyer lift is used for clients who are weak or very overweight. Choice **c** is incorrect; it is usually not necessary to have three persons to conduct a proper transfer. Choice **d** is incorrect; special mattresses are usually designed to prevent pressure sores.

47. c. Self-esteem promotes wellness. Dressing improves self-esteem for all clients—most residents want to be as independent as possible. All residents are entitled to privacy.

48. c. A *delusion* is a faulty belief. A *hallucination* is a faulty sensory perception, and seeing demons is a faulty visual perception. Feeling bugs crawling on one's skin is a faulty tactile perception. Hearing voices is a faulty auditory perception.

49. d. Constantly reminding the client about loss will only depress him. Labeling items helps reinforce the name of the items. Calendars and clocks help orient the client to day and time. Using familiar items helps the client know which room is his.

50. a. All patients need to feel wanted and to share their feelings with another person. This is normal behavior. Choice **b** is incorrect; there is no reason why a client with muscular dystrophy should feel hopeless about relationships. Choice **c** is incorrect; having a relationship is realistic for persons with physical disabilities. Choice **d** is incorrect; this is a normal feeling, not a sign of confusion.

51. d. The client has a right to privacy. Choice **a** is incorrect; clients have a right to appropriately express their sexuality. Choice **b** is incorrect; masturbation is a normal behavior, and the client should not have to explain why he is masturbating in his bathroom. Choice **c** is incorrect; there is no need to report this normal behavior to the charge nurse.

52. c. Standard precautions must be used during postmortem care. Wearing gloves is mandatory. The body continues to be infectious following death. It is not required that a family member be present during postmortem care. However, in some cultures, family members clean and prepare the body for what lies ahead. It is helpful to have a coworker assist in postmortem care, but not required. It is not the nurse aide's role to contact the funeral director.

53. a. The last sense to leave is hearing. Speak with kindness and be aware of what you say. Unconscious clients are not able to move on their own and are at risk for decubiti. Unconscious patients may have dry skin.

54. c. The response reflects confidentiality for all clients as well as an appropriate, unoffensive response to the roommate. Choice **a** is incorrect; saying that it is really nothing for you to worry about is condescending to the roommate. Choice **b** is incorrect; the nurse aide does not directly consult with the doctor, and she cannot tell the roommate about the client's condition because of confidentiality. Choice **d** is incorrect; the doctor cannot tell the roommate about the client either, and the nurse aide should not instruct the roommate to call.

55. c. The plan assures that nursing care is consistent with the patient's needs, and progresses toward self-care. The nursing diagnosis is part of the care plan. The diagnosis states the patient's problem. Both short- and long-term goals and scheduled appointments are part of the care plan and are part of the planning phase.

56. d. Report all changes to the charge nurse, regardless of the client's age. The nurse aide is not allowed to give ear drops. Placing a warm cloth on the baby's ear is a treatment and should not be done by the nurse aide without instruction. The baby is in pain and not hungry.

57. a. Listening carefully to the client's needs encourages communication and builds trust. Choice **b** is incorrect; if the person cannot hear you over the call bell system, answer the call in person. Choice **c** is incorrect; the call bell should never be unplugged, and the client should always have access to the call bell. Unplugging it can be seen as abuse. Choice **d** is incorrect; the nurse aide does not report to the supervisor, and the client is not being uncooperative. Clients may use the call system excessively when they are scared or lonely.

58. d. Mental status exams are not performed by nurse aides. Choice **a** is incorrect; the client has a right to privacy. Choice **b** is incorrect; the nurse aide should ensure that the water is not too hot so that the client does not get burned. Choice **c** is incorrect; the nurse aide should have all supplies before giving the client her bath because the nurse aide cannot leave the client alone once the bath begins.

59. d. Dietary supplements are high in necessary vitamins and minerals. Vitamins are considered a medication and therefore cannot be given by the nurse aide. A tube feeding requires a physician's order. Clear broth does not have adequate nutrition.

60. c. In death, the body shuts down, and there are no vital signs. Convulsions are not always a sign of death, nor are they always seen at the time of death. Loss of consciousness and lack of response do not necessarily mean impending death.

61. a. It is important to accommodate the religious beliefs of the client. It is not the nurse aide's role to call a priest and ask for dispensation, and the nurse aide should not interpret the client's religious beliefs for him. It is important for the client's religion that he not eat meat on that specific day.

62. c. It is important to accommodate the client's cultural and religious beliefs in her healthcare regimen. This begins with assessing the client's cultural and religious needs. The nurse aide does not call the dietician; the nurse performs this function. The nurse aide also does not need to report this to the charge nurse, unless it will cause problems for the client. Telling the client she must eat her food deprives her of her right to follow her religious beliefs.

63. b. Anything told in confidence cannot be revealed, unless what was said will result in harm to the client or someone else.

64. b. All incidents must be described exactly as observed. The nurse aide should not be subjective about the incident. Client falls need to be reported immediately, even if this is not the nurse aide's client. The nurse aide needs to report exactly what she sees and not add any additional information.

65. b. Nurse aides should not accept monetary gifts from clients and their families. Ethically, the nurse aide should not accept it, even to be polite. While using the money for the client is admirable, the nurse aide should not take money from a client. There is no need to report this to the charge nurse.

66. b. Residents have a right to be alone to grieve after the death of a loved one. Keeping busy to keep her mind off the loss disallows the resident to grieve properly. The resident should be allowed to meet other men when she is ready to do so. Crying is a normal part of grieving.

67. a. Residents can refuse treatment or therapy because of the Patient's Bill of Rights. Residents do not need their physician's permission to refuse treatment. They should be able to take part in their treatment planning, which includes their right to refuse treatments.

68. c. All clients are treated according to the Patient's Bill of Rights. State hospital and physicians' associations do not determine client rights. The Caregiver Bill of Rights refers to caregivers, not clients.

69. b. All clients have the right to privacy and should be properly covered at all times. Choice **a** is incorrect; the right to confidentiality means the client's information remains confidential. Choice **c** is incorrect; there is no specific right to nursing care plans; however, clients have a right to considerate and respectful care. Choice **d** is incorrect. The client has a right to make decisions about her care and to refuse a recommended treatment.

70. c. The identification of healthcare workers allows the patient to know the identity of physicians, nurses, and others involved in their care. An example of *considerate and respectful care* would be the nurse allowing a resident to grieve after the resident learned of the death of her husband. An example of the *right to privacy* is the nurse keeping the curtains closed when bathing the client. The patient has the right to know how the hospital settles disputes, what the hospital charges, and the payment options.

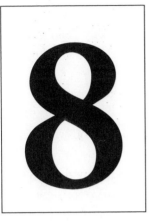

CHAPTER

NURSING ASSISTANT/NURSE AIDE PRACTICAL SKILLS EXAM

CHAPTER SUMMARY

For most states' certification requirements, you will be asked to complete a performance evaluation—a hands-on test of your practical skills as well as a written or oral exam. This chapter gives a sample of the variety of job tasks you will be asked to perform.

As previously noted, state requirements vary, and this chapter looks at the probable scenario. In order to be certified as a nursing assistant, you will be asked to perform five job-related skills. Handwashing will most likely be one of the skills, while the other four will be randomly selected from a list of nurse aide skills. A measurement skill, such as measuring urinary output, will probably be included in these remaining four skills, and you will be required to record that measurement. You will perform these skills in a hospital/nursing home-like setting while being observed by the evaluator. A volunteer will act as the client.

Each skill is broken down into steps, and some of these are critical steps that must be completed to pass the skill. However, you must also successfully complete an adequate number of steps to pass each skill, and you must pass all five skills to pass the entire skills exam. You will be expected to know and perform these steps; directions will not be provided.

Equipment will be provided, and you may not be allowed to use your own equipment. The evaluator will not give you instructions or answer any questions during the skill performance, so ask questions before you begin. If you think you made a mistake during a skill performance, tell the evaluator at that time. You will be allowed to correct the steps that you did incorrectly—one time. There are some exceptions to this, and some corrections will not receive credit. Also, once you begin a new skill, you will not be allowed to go back and redo a previous one.

This chapter provides you with several job-related skills you might be asked to perform: handwashing; counting the radial pulse; counting respirations; measuring blood pressure; donning and removing gown and gloves, or Personal Protective Equipment (PPE); measuring urinary output; positioning on side; and transferring from bed to wheelchair. Each skill list contains tips and evaluation criteria. Practice these skills, using a friend or family member as your client, and review the skills list after you are done to make sure you did not miss any steps. You should utilize your nurse aide textbook to practice other job-related skills, especially those in which you need improvement. You should also contact your state's nurse aide registry to acquire a list of testable skills and expected steps. The registry office will be able to tell you how much time is allowed for each skill performance.

Practice, practice, practice. Have a nurse or nurse aide observe you with the skill step-list in hand to make sure you are performing the skills correctly, step-by-step. Practice first for accuracy. Once you know you can perform the steps correctly, practice to ensure that you can complete the skills in the required time frame.

Sample Skill: Handwashing

Tips:

1. Handwashing is the single most important method of preventing the spread of infection.
2. When washing your hands, make sure to clean under the fingernails, and between the fingers.
3. Do not wear nail polish or artificial nails for the skills exam, and keep your nails trimmed short. Avoid wearing rings and bracelets.
4. Do not touch the inside of the sink at any time during handwashing.

Evaluation Criteria

- Introduce yourself and address the client by title and surname.
- Make sure paper towels are within reach and ready to use—you do not want to touch the "dirty" paper towel container with your freshly cleaned hands.
- Turn on the water at the sink—be careful, no splashing.
- Wet your hands and wrists thoroughly.
- Apply soap.
- Lather and rub fingers, hands, and wrists for at least 15 seconds.
- Clean your fingernails by rubbing the tips of your fingers against the palm of the opposite hand.
- Rinse fingers, hands, and wrists thoroughly; keep your hands lower than your elbows and your fingertips pointed down.
- Dry hands thoroughly with clean paper towel and dispose of paper towel. Dispose of paper towel in a waste container without contaminating yourself.
- Turn off the faucet with another clean paper towel, and dispose of that paper towel in a waste container without contaminating yourself.

Sample Skill: Radial Pulse

Tips:

1. You should count the radial pulse for one full minute. Bring a watch with a second hand.
2. Do not use your thumb to count the pulse.

Evaluation Criteria

- Introduce yourself and address the client by title and surname.
- Wash your hands (see the Handwashing section).
- Explain the procedure to the client, speaking in a clear, slow manner. Make sure to maintain eye contact whenever possible.
- Locate the client's radial pulse by placing two fingers over the radial artery (on the inside of the wrist).
- Count the pulse for a full minute.

- Wash your hands (see the Handwashing section).
- Record the client's pulse rate.

Sample Skill: Respirations

Tips:

1. The respiratory rate may be affected by fever, pain, fear, disease, and other factors.
2. People can control their respirations to some extent (e.g., holding one's breath).
3. Do not tell the client that you are measuring her respiratory rate, because that will affect the reading. Instead, take it immediately after you measure her radial pulse. This is one time it is acceptable to perform a task without telling the client what you are going to do.
4. Count respirations by watching the rise and fall of the chest, and/or by placing your hand against the person's chest and feeling for the rise and fall.

Evaluation Criteria

- Introduce yourself and address the client by title and surname.
- Wash your hands (see the Handwashing section).
- Explain the procedure to the client, speaking in a clear, slow manner. Make sure to maintain eye contact whenever possible.
- Count respirations for a full minute.
- Wash your hands (see the Handwashing section).
- Record the client's respiratory rate.

Sample Skill: Blood Pressure

Tips:

1. The systolic pressure is the top number and is pressure caused when the heart muscle contracts.
2. The diastolic pressure is the lower number and is created when the heart muscle relaxes.

3. If you cannot find the brachial artery, have the client hyperextend his arm and try again.
4. Use the correct size cuff, or the blood pressure measurement will not be accurate.

Evaluation Criteria

- Introduce yourself and address the client by title and surname.
- Wash your hands (see the Handwashing section).
- Explain the procedure to the client, speaking in a clear, slow manner. Make sure to maintain eye contact whenever possible.
- Clean ear pieces and diaphragm/bell of stethoscope with an alcohol wipe.
- Position client's arm with the palm up and upper arm exposed.
- Find the brachial artery at the bend of the elbow, on the inner aspect of the arm.
- Place the correct size blood pressure cuff snugly on the client's upper arm with the arrow over the brachial artery.
- Locate the radial pulse (see the Radial Pulse section).
- Inflate the cuff to no more than 30 mm Hg more than where the pulse is felt.
- Deflate the cuff.
- Locate the brachial artery again, using your fingertips.
- Put the stethoscope in your ears and place the diaphragm/bell over the brachial artery.
- Inflate the cuff to no more than 30 mm Hg more than where the pulse is felt.
- Deflate cuff slowly and note the first sound that you hear (systolic).
- Note the last sound you hear (diastolic).
- Remove the cuff.
- Wash hands (see the Handwashing section).
- Record blood pressure reading, both systolic and diastolic.

Sample Skill: Measuring Urinary Output

Tips:

1. Some people who are critically ill need to have their urinary output measured hourly.
2. If a client uses the regular toilet, the client can use a "commode hat" to collect the urine for measuring.
3. Make sure to hold the measuring container at eye level to determine the amount.

Evaluation Criteria

- Introduce yourself and address the client by title and surname.
- Wash your hands (see the Handwashing section).
- Explain the procedure to the client, speaking in a clear, slow manner. Make sure to maintain eye contact whenever possible.
- Put on clean gloves before touching the bedpan.
- Pour the contents of the bedpan into a measuring container. Do not spill or splash urine.
- Measure urine at eye level with the container securely placed on a flat surface.
- After measuring urine, empty the measuring container.
- Rinse the measuring container and pour rinse contents into the toilet.
- Rinse the bedpan and pour rinse contents into the toilet.
- Remove gloves. Dispose of gloves in a waste container without contaminating yourself.
- Wash hands (see the Handwashing section).
- Record urine output.

Sample Skill: Positioning on Side (Lateral Position)

Tips:

1. Make sure you have supportive devices ready before positioning client.
2. The lateral position is used for people with back pain, those in casts, and those who cannot reposition themselves.

Evaluation Criteria

- Introduce yourself and address the client by title and surname.
- Wash your hands (see the Handwashing section).
- Explain the procedure to the client, speaking in a clear, slow manner. Make sure to maintain eye contact whenever possible.
- Provide privacy by closing the curtain or door.
- Lower the head of the bed.
- Raise side rail on the side toward which the client will be turned.
- Slowly roll client as one unit onto his side, toward the raised side rail.
- Place a pillow under his head for support.
- Make sure client is not lying on the arm that is on the bed, and support the top arm with a supportive device.
- Place supportive device behind the client's back.
- Flex the client's top knee and place supportive device between the client's legs; make sure the knee and ankle are supported.
- Lower the bed.
- Make sure the call bell is within reach.
- Wash hands (see the Handwashing section).

Sample Skill: Personal Protective Equipment (PPE)— Donning and Removing Gown and Gloves

Tips:

1. PPE includes gowns, gloves, masks, and protective eyewear.
2. Gloves must be intact and fit properly.
3. If you are allergic to latex, use gloves made from another synthetic material.
4. If you touch a contaminated surface with your gloves, your gloves become contaminated.
5. Gowns are used when you are likely to soil your uniform with bodily fluids and for certain types of isolation.

Evaluation Criteria

- Introduce yourself and address the client by title and surname.
- Wash your hands (see the Handwashing section).

Donning the gown and gloves

- Unfold gown.
- With back opening of gown facing you, place arms through each of the sleeves.
- Fasten the neck ties.
- Secure the gown at your waist, and make sure your clothing is covered as much as possible.
- Put on gloves, making sure the cuffs of the gloves overlap the cuffs of the gown.

Removing the gown and gloves.

- Use one gloved hand to remove the opposite glove at the palm.
- Slip the fingers from your ungloved hand under the cuff of the remaining glove and remove the glove, turning it inside out as you proceed.
- Dispose of gloves in a waste container without contaminating yourself.
- Untie the gown at the neck and waist.

- Remove the gown without touching the outside of the gown.
- Hold the gown away from your body and turn it inward to keep it inside out.
- Dispose of gown in a waste container without contaminating yourself.
- Wash hands (see the Handwashing section).

Sample Skill: Transferring Client from Bed to Wheelchair

Tips:

1. A transfer belt is used to assist weak or unsteady persons with transferring, walking, and standing. Many facilities require nurse aides to use these when transferring clients.
2. Always plan in advance when transferring clients. Know your client's specific limitations.
3. Wheelchairs should be checked to make sure they have no broken or missing parts.
4. Make sure to lock the brakes before transferring clients into and out of wheelchairs.

Evaluation Criteria

- Introduce yourself and address the client by title and surname.
- Wash your hands (see the Handwashing section).
- Explain the procedure to the client, speaking in a clear, slow manner. Make sure to maintain eye contact whenever possible.
- Provide privacy by pulling the curtain or shutting the door.
- Position the wheelchair at the side of the bed, facing the foot of the bed.
- Make sure footrests are removed or folded up.
- Make sure to lock the wheelchair brakes.
- Assist the client into a sitting position with her feet flat on the floor. Make sure the client is wearing shoes before the client attempts to stand.
- Securely apply the transfer belt over the client's clothing before assisting her to stand.

- Instruct the client on the transfer process and provide her with a signal for when to begin standing (e.g., "Stand on three.").
- Stand facing the client during transfer.
- Count to three to alert the client to begin standing.
- On "three," slowly help the client to stand by grasping the transfer belt on both sides with an upward grasp. Maintain the stability of the client's legs.
- Assist the client to turn to stand in front of the wheelchair, making sure her legs are against the wheelchair.

- Lower the client into the wheelchair.
- Position the client so that her hips touch the back of the chair, assuring that she is not sitting on any objects that may cause pressure to her skin.
- Remove the transfer belt.
- Position footrests in the down position and assist the client in placing her feet on them.
- Make sure the client's call bell is within reach.
- Wash hands (see the Handwashing section).

9 ▶ CERTIFICATION REQUIREMENTS AND TRENDS

CHAPTER SUMMARY

This chapter provides an overview of state certification and licensing requirements for nursing assistants. It will also help you keep abreast of the trends—what's new in healthcare certification.

Although there is no national organization for the certification of nursing assistants, there is a certification exam that is utilized by several states. The National Nurse Aide Assessment Program (NNAAP) is the largest nursing assistant certification examination in the United States. The National Council of State Boards of Nursing (NCSBN) develops the examination program and administers it with a test service.

State Certification and Training

Since OBRA '87 (Omnibus Budget Reconciliation Act of 1987) was passed, the federal government has been setting regulations and creating standards for the quality of nursing home care. Specific guidelines and standards were prescribed—one major change was the training and testing of nursing assistants/nurse aides. In many states, nurse aides are required to go through a minimum of 75 hours of training approved by the federal government to be certified. Most programs are between 75 and 150 hours and vary by state. Some states have created their own standards for nursing assistants. These standards include the minimum training requirements as well as a written exam of multiple-choice questions and clinical/practical evaluations. Most healthcare facilities now require nurse aides to have a high school diploma or GED and pass a state-approved program. Nurse aides completing these programs must obtain certification within four months of being hired at a healthcare facility. Once you pass the written exam, you will be placed on your state's registry for nurse aides. Your certification is then valid for 24 months. After being certified, CNAs are usually required to earn 12 continuing-education credits annually, often through inservice training.

Eligibility for Certification

Most states have multiple eligibility options to meet the needs of nursing assistants with various backgrounds. The following list represents most types of eligibility, but you should check with your state's nurse aide registry for its requirements.

- New Nursing Assistants are persons who have never been certified as a nursing assistant/nurse aide. These candidates must complete a state-approved nursing assistant education program prior to taking the exam.
- Nursing Students include those who have successfully completed a nursing fundamentals course through a state-approved nursing program within one year of applying to take the examination, and those who have successfully completed the fundamentals course and are currently enrolled in a nursing program.
- Graduate Nurses are nurses who graduated from a state-approved nursing program and who are waiting to take the state nursing licensing examination.
- Foreign Graduate Nurses graduated a nursing program in a foreign country and are currently nurses in that country.

- Nursing Assistants in another state can apply for reciprocity. These are persons currently certified as a nurse aide in another state and listed in that other state's nurse aide registry (and usually who have not had their certificate revoked in any state or been listed on any state's nurse aide abuse registry).
- Military Nurse Aides have equivalent nurse aide training and experience in a military service.
- Lapsed or Expired Certification pertains to persons who are applying back to the state in which they were originally certified and whose certification has lapsed or expired (and usually who have not had their certificate revoked in any state or been listed on any state's nurse aide abuse registry).

Training Programs

Nursing assistant training programs prepare students for employment as nursing assistants in hospitals, long-term-care facilities, hospices, home-health agencies, and other healthcare agencies. Programs average a total of 120 hours of combined classroom and clinical education, allowing those who complete the program to sit for the certification exam.

Content is similar from one program to the next and typically includes:

- Overview of the Healthcare System
- The Healthcare Team
- The Role of the Nursing Assistant
- Working with Coworkers and Supervisors
- Work Ethics
- Problem Solving and Conflict Management
- Client and Resident Rights
- Violations of Criminal and Civil Law
- Medical Terminology
- Effective Communications
- Human Growth and Development
- The Human Body and Common Disorders:
  - The Integumentary System (Skin, Hair, and Nails)
  - The Respiratory System

- The Cardiovascular System
- The Digestive System
- The Endocrine System
- The Hematologic System
- The Musculoskeletal System
- The Nervous System
- The Sensory System
- The Immunologic System
- Admissions and Discharges
- Infection Control
- Client Safety and Restraint
- Workplace Safety
- Positioning
- Nutrition and Feeding
- Urinary and Bowel Elimination
- Basic First Aid
- Basic Emergency Care
- Death and Dying
- Specific Populations
  - Older Adults
  - Children
  - Mothers and Newborns
  - Persons with Disabilities
  - Persons with Mental Illness
  - Surgical Clients
  - Home-Health Clients
  - Hospice Clients

Nursing assistant students also learn and practice job-related skills:

- Handwashing and Hand Hygiene
- Vital Signs: Blood Pressure, Temperature, Pulse, and Respiration
- Measuring Height and Weight
- Oral Care
- Denture Care
- Fingernail Care
- Foot Care
- Perineal Care
- Bed Baths
- Applying Knee-High Stockings

- Dressing Clients with One-Sided Weakness
- Feeding Clients
- Measuring Urinary Output
- Urinary Catheter Care
- Ostomy Care
- Administering Enemas
- Administering Hot and Cold Applications
- Assisting with Dressing Changes
- Ambulating Clients Using a Transfer Belt
- Positioning Clients
- Transferring Clients from Bed to Wheelchair (Wheelchair to Bed)
- Passive Range of Motion Exercises
- Using Personal Protective Equipment
- Postmortem Care

A major part of the job of being a CNA involves being able to manipulate patients physically in order to clean them and help them change their clothes, exercise, or use the bathroom. The clinical part of the training programs helps to determine if a student is capable of performing these tasks.

Training programs are given in a number of settings, including both public and private vocational-technical schools, community colleges, public-health agencies, and for-profit and not-for-profit healthcare agencies, such as visiting nurse associations. Since hands-on clinical experience is usually required, schools that do not have their own healthcare services often affiliate with a healthcare facility. Then the course work is given in the school and the clinical work is performed in the healthcare facility or in a home setting served by a healthcare agency.

In the states that require certification, there are usually a large number of locations that offer training programs. In Illinois, for example, there are some 300 approved CNA training programs. Agencies that offer training programs often hire the people they have trained, so they are good places to sign up for a training program that may lead to a job offer when you complete the course.

Each program has its own admission requirements. But, like program content, requirements tend to be similar among programs:

- minimum age of 16 or 18 years, depending on program
- completion of COMPASS, ACT, or ASSET test before entering program (these test your verbal, reading, and numerical skills); minimum scores are set by the training program.
- ability to pass a national criminal background check and a caregiver background check (Certain convictions may limit a student's ability to participate in clinical experiences or be employed in healthcare facilities. Examples include convictions related to drugs, theft, violence, disorderly conduct, domestic abuse, theft, and fraud.)
- physical exam (certain vaccinations may be required)

Other possible requirements:

- high school diploma or GED
- health insurance
- ability to lift heavy weight and stand for long periods

Exams

Training programs usually conclude with a written (or oral) examination that determines whether the student is qualified to receive certification. Some institutions that offer training make up their own examinations, while others may use an exam prepared by a company that specializes in developing tests. Tests typically range from 50 to 150 questions and are in sections that relate directly to the subject areas covered in the training, such as patient-care procedures, emergency procedures, or observation and charting. Usually a candidate must achieve a passing grade in each of the sections, and not just overall, in order to qualify for certification.

Why Certification?

The main reason behind the trend to CNA certification is the growth of home healthcare. Home-based healthcare has been on the increase because of cost-saving measures in the health industry: Patients are being encouraged to leave relatively expensive hospital-based care to complete their recuperations in lower-cost alternative settings, including short-term- and long-term-care facilities, as well as the home. Nursing assistants work in a wide variety of healthcare settings, including skilled-nursing facilities, doctors' offices, hospices, board-and-care retirement facilities, acute-care hospitals, clinics, rehabilitation hospitals, psychiatric hospitals, facilities for the developmentally disabled, and daycare facilities. But the delivery of services in patient homes is what has increased awareness on the part of state and national authorities, leading to the increase of requirements for certification.

Certification offers assurance that nursing assistants, who have such immediate, important, and intimate contact with elderly or disabled persons, have been properly trained to deal with the many and varied tasks they will have to perform. It is also important to healthcare agencies that, in addition to providing care for the patient, CNAs be able to acknowledge the psychosocial needs of the patient's family. The federal government, which is often the funding source for home healthcare under the Medicare program, also wants to know that its funds are being spent for high-quality services.

Emphasis on Interpersonal Skills

While it has always been important for healthcare professionals of all kinds to be able to make patients feel safe and comfortable, these skills become even more crucial when care is being delivered in the patient's own home or in long-term care. Thus, many training programs are now emphasizing interpersonal skills more than ever before. In the sample training programs shown earlier in this chapter, you can see that interpersonal skills, such as Effective Communication and Client and Resident Rights, are emphasized.

Combining CNA and Home Health Aide Certification

The trend to certification is also spurred by the fact that the training programs for nursing assistants typically include the training requirements for the job of home-health aide (HHA), as well. HHA training follows a federally mandated 75-hour curriculum. The federal mandate is there because home-health agencies are eligible for Medicare funds for the services they provide to the elderly.

Since CNAs can perform medical tasks beyond what HHAs are trained to do, someone who has training and certification in both job categories is obviously of greater value to the agency doing the hiring. The employer is better off hiring one person who can perform two different jobs, even if that one person's salary is a little higher than that of a person with one certification.

The home-health aide profession is growing faster than average and should continue growing. The reason for this is the increased need for home care of the elderly—patients are being moved out of hospitals and nursing homes to lower healthcare costs. In 2008, more than 1.7 million people were employed as home-health aides and most were employed in home-health agencies, nursing facilities, hospitals, visiting-nurse associations, residential-care facilities, and temporary-help firms. Full-time aides work about 40 hours per week, while many aides work part time. The actual job can be difficult both physically and emotionally; it includes a good portion of standing, lifting, changing bed linens, and dealing with uncooperative clients. Generally, a home-health aide works independently and with a variety of patients. Supervisors visit sporadically, and the aide is always given explicit instructions pertaining to schedule and patient care.

In Massachusetts, persons entering home-health aide programs are often encouraged to undergo dual training and become CNAs in order to improve their employment opportunities.

In some states, such as Illinois, people who want to become home-health aides are required to take the same training program as CNAs. The HHA training is included within the program as part of the CNA training. As a result, the certification that follows the successful completion of the CNA training and the passage of the written competency examination serves as a dual certification for home-health aides as well.

The good news for people who want to become nursing assistants is that the growth of healthcare in alternative settings ensures that workers will be needed. CNAs can look forward to good job prospects for the foreseeable future.

10 ▶ IMPORTANT RESOURCES

CHAPTER SUMMARY

This chapter identifies numerous healthcare organizations and services—potentially valuable resources in your search for the right job.

f you're just getting started on your new healthcare career—or if you're wondering how you can go about finding a job—the resources listed in this chapter can give you valuable background information. Included here are lists of professional organizations, directories, placement services, and home-care organizations.

Professional Associations

Professional associations are made up of experts in the nursing field. Both members and the people who run these organizations are actively working in and on the behalf of, the fields they represent. Above all, they are great sources of information on possible careers, education and training programs, and professional requirements such as certification and licensure. In most cases, if these folks don't have the information you need, they can tell you who will.

In addition, many professional associations offer job placement or referral services. Many publish newsletters, magazines, books, and other publications, as well as multimedia products such as videos and CD-ROMs.

Many also sponsor seminars, workshops, and other educational forums. All of these efforts can help interested individuals keep up on current happenings in a given field.

Nursing Assistant Organizations

National Association of Health Care Assistants
501 E. 15th St.
Joplin, MO 64804
Phone: 800-784-6049
Fax: 417-623-2230
Website: www.nahcacares.org

National Network of Career Nursing Assistants
Website: www.cna-network.org

Nursing Assistant Resources
Website: www.nursingassistants.net

National Nursing Organizations

Academy of Medical-Surgical Nurses
E. Holly Ave., Box 56
Pitman, NJ 08071
Phone: 866-877-2676
Website: www.medsurgnurse.org

Air & Surface Transport Nurses Association
7995 E. Prentice Ave., Ste. 100
Greenwood Village, CO 80111
Phone: 303-770-1614/800-897-NFNA (6362)
Website: www.astna.org

American Academy of Ambulatory Care Nursing
E. Holly Ave., Box 56
Pitman, NJ 08071
Phone: 800-262-6877
Website: www.aaacn.org

American Assembly for Men in Nursing
P.O. Box 130220
Birmingham, AL 35213
Phone: 205-956-0146
Website: www.aamn.org

American Association of Critical-Care Nurses
101 Columbia
Aliso Viejo, CA 92656
Phone: 949-362-2050
Website: www.aacn.org

American Association of Diabetes Educators
200 W. Madison St., Ste. 800
Chicago, IL 60606
Phone: 800-338-3633
Website: www.aadenet.org

American Association of Legal Nurse Consultants
401 N. Michigan Ave.
Chicago, IL 60611
Phone: 877-402-2562
Website: www.aalnc.org

American Association of Neuroscience Nurses
4700 W. Lake Ave.
Glenview, IL 60025
Phone: 888-557-2266
Website: www.aann.org

American Association of Nurse Anesthetists
222 S. Prospect Ave.
Park Ridge, IL 60068
Phone: 847-692-7050
Website: www.aana.com

American Association of Nurse Attorneys
P.O. Box 14218
Lenexa, KS 66285-4218
Toll-Free: 877-538-2262
Website: www.taana.org

American Association of Occupational Health Nurses
7794 Grow Dr.
Pensacola, FL 32514
Phone: 850-474-6963/800-241-8014
Fax: 850-484-8762
Website: www.aaohn.org

American College of Nurse Midwives
8403 Colesville Rd., Ste. 1550
Silver Spring, MD 20910
Phone: 240-485-1800
Website: www.midwife.org

American Holistic Nurses' Association
323 N. San Francisco St., Ste. 201
Flagstaff, AZ 86001
Phone: 800-278-2462
Website: www.ahna.org

American Nephrology Nurses' Association
E. Holly Ave., Box 56
Pitman, NJ 08071
Phone: 888-600-2662
Website: www.annanurse.org

American Nurses Association
8515 Georgia Ave., Ste. 400
Silver Spring, MD 20910
Phone: 800-274-4ANA (4262)
Website: www.nursingworld.org

American Organization of Nurse Executives
155 N. Wacker Dr., Ste. 400
Chicago, IL 60606
Phone: 312-422-2800
Website: www.aone.org

American Psychiatric Nurses Association
1555 Wilson Blvd., Ste. 530
Arlington, VA 22209
Phone: 866-243-2443
Website: www.apna.org

American Public Health Association
800 I St., NW
Washington, DC 20001
Phone: 202-777-APHA (2742)
Website: www.apha.org

American Society of Ophthalmic Registered Nurses
P.O. Box 193030
San Francisco, CA 94119
Phone: 415-561-8513
Website: www.asorn.org

American Society of Pain Management Nurses
P.O. Box 15473
Lenexa, KS 66285-5473
Phone: 888-34ASPMN (342-7766)
Website: www.aspmn.org

American Society of Perianesthesia Nurses
90 Frontage Rd.
Cherry Hill, NJ 08034-1424
Phone: 877-737-9696
Fax: 856-616-9601
Website: www.aspan.org

American Society of Plastic and Reconstructive/ Surgical Nurses
500 Cummings Center, Ste. 4550
Beverly, MA 01915
Phone: 877-337-9315
Website: www.aspsn.org

Association for Radiologic & Imaging Nursing
7794 Grow Dr.
Pensacola, FL 32514
Phone: 866-486-2762
Website: www.arinursing.org

Association of Community Health Nurse Educators
10200 W. 44th Ave., Ste. 304
Wheat Ridge, CO 80033
Phone: 303-422-0769
Website: www.achne.org

Association of Occupational Health Professionals
109 VIP Dr., Ste. 220
Wexford, PA 15090
Phone: 800-362-4347
Website: www.aohp.org

Association of Pediatric Hematology/ Oncology Nurses
4700 W. Lake Ave.
Glenview, IL 60025
Phone: 847-375-4724
Website: www.apon.org

Association of periOperative Registered Nurses
2170 S. Parker Rd., Ste. 400
Denver, CO 80231
Phone: 800-755-2676
Website: www.aorn.org

Association of Nurses in AIDS Care
3538 Ridgewood Rd.
Akron, OH 44333
Phone: 800-260-6780
Website: www.anacnet.org

Association of Rehabilitation Nurses
4700 W. Lake Ave.
Glenview, IL 60025
Phone: 800-229-7530
Website: www.rehabnurse.org

Association of Women's Health, Obstetric and Neonatal Nurses
2000 L St., NW, Ste. 740
Washington, DC 20036
Phone: 800-673-8499
Website: www.awhonn.org

Association for Professionals in Infection Control and Epidemiology
1275 K St. NW, Ste. 1000
Washington, DC, 20005
Phone: 202-789-1890
Website: www.apic.org

Dermatology Nurses' Association
15000 Commerce Pkwy., Ste. C
Mt. Laurel, NJ 08054
Phone: 800-454-4362
Website: www.dnanurse.org

Developmental Disabilities Nurses Association
P.O. Box 536489
Orlando, FL 32853
Phone: 800-888-6733
Website: www.ddna.org

Emergency Nurses Association
915 Lee St.
Des Plaines, IL 60016
Phone: 800-900-9659
Website: www.ena.org

Endocrine Society
8401 Connecticut Ave., Ste. 900
Chevy Chase, MD 20815-5817
Phone: 301-941-0200
Website: www.endo-society.org

Hospice and Palliative Nurses Association
One Penn Center W., Ste. 229
Pittsburgh, PA 15276
Phone: 412-787-9301
Website: www.hpna.org

Infusion Nurses Society
315 Norwood Park S.
Norwood, MA 02062
Phone: 781-440-9408
Website: www.ins1.org

International Association of Forensic Nurses
1517 Ritchie Hwy., Ste. 208
Arnold, MD 21012
Phone: 410-626-7805
Website: www.iafn.org

International Nurses Society on Addictions
P.O. Box 163635
Columbus, OH 43216
Phone: 877-646-8672
Website: www.intnsa.org

International Organization of Multiple Sclerosis Nurses
P.O. Box 450
Teaneck, NJ 07666
Phone: 201-487-1050
Website: www.iomsn.org

International Society of Nurses in Genetics
461 Cochran Rd.
Box 246
Pittsburgh, PA 15528
Phone: 414-344-1414
Website: www.isong.org

National Association for Associate Degree Nursing
7794 Grow Dr.
Pensacola, FL 32514
Phone: 877-966-6236
Website: www.noadn.org

National Association for Home Care and Hospice
228 Seventh St., SE
Washington, DC 20003
Phone: 202-547-7424
Website: www.nahc.org

National Association for Practical Nurse Education and Service
1940 Duke St., Ste. 200
Alexandria, VA 22314
Phone: 703-933-1003
Website: www.napnes.org

National Association of Clinical Nurse Specialists
100 N. 20th St., 4th Fl.
Philadelphia, PA 19103
Phone: 215-320-3881
Website: www.nacns.org

National Association of Hispanic Nurses
1455 Pennsylvania Ave., NW, Ste. 400
Washington, DC 20004
Phone: 202-387-2477
Website: www.thehispanicnurses.org

National Association of Nurse Massage Therapists
28 Lowry Dr.
P.O. Box 232
West Milton, OH 45383
Phone: 800-262-4017
Website: www.nanmt.org

National Association of Nurse Practitioners in Women's Health
505 C St., NE
Washington, DC 20002
Phone: 202-543-9693
Website: www.npwh.org

National Association of Orthopedic Nurses
401 N. Michigan Ave., Ste. 2200
Chicago, IL 60611
Phone: 800-289-6266
Website: www.orthonurse.org

National Association of Pediatric Nurse Practitioners
20 Brace Rd., Ste. 200
Cherry Hill, NJ 08034
Phone: 856-857-9700
Website: www.napnap.org

National Association of School Nurses
8484 Georgia Ave., Ste. 420
Silver Spring, MD 20910
Phone: 240-821-1130
Website: www.nasn.org

National Black Nurses Association
8630 Fenton St., Ste. 330
Silver Spring, MD 20910
Phone: 301-589-3200
Website: www.nbna.org

National Federation of Licensed Practical Nurses
111 W. Main St., Ste. 100
Garner, NC 27529
Phone: 919-779-0046
Website: www.nflpn.org

National Gerontological Nurses Association
3493 Lansdowne Dr., Ste. 2
Lexington, KY 40517
Phone: 859-977-7453
Website: www.ngna.org

National League for Nursing
61 Broadway, 33rd Fl.
New York, NY 10006
Phone: 800-669-1656
Website: www.nln.org

National Student Nurses' Association
45 Main St., Ste. 606
Brooklyn, NY 11201
Phone: 718-210-0705
Website: www.nsna.org

North American Nursing Diagnosis Association
P.O. Box 157
Kaukauna, WI 54130
Phone: 920-344-8670
Website: www.nanda.org

Nursing Division of the American Association of Mental Retardation
501 3rd St., NW Ste. 200
Washington, DC 20001
Phone: 800-424-3688
Website: www.aamr.org

Oncology Nursing Society
125 Enterprise Dr.
Pittsburgh, PA 15275
Phone: 866-257-4ONS (4667)
Website: www.ons.org

Respiratory Nursing Society
Box 980567
Richmond, VA 23298
Website: www.respiratorynursingsociety.org

Society for Vascular Nursing
100 Cummings Ctr., Ste. 124 A
Beverly, MA 01915
Phone: 888-536-4786/978-927-7800
Fax: 978-927-7827
Website: www.svnnet.org

Society of Gastroenterology Nurses and Associates
401 N. Michigan Ave.
Chicago, IL 60611
Phone: 800-245-7462
Website: www.sgna.org

Society of Otorhinolaryngology and Head-Neck Nurses
207 Downing St.
New Smyrna Beach, FL 32168
Phone: 386-428-1695
Website: www.sohnnurse.com

Society of Pediatric Nurses
7044 S. 13th St.
Oak Creek, WI 53154
Phone: 414-908-4950
Website: www.pedsnurses.org

Society of Urologic Nurses and Associates
E. Holly Ave., Box 56
Pitman, NJ 08071
Phone: 888-827-7862
Website: www.suna.org

Transcultural Nursing Society
Madonna University
36600 Schoolcraft Rd.
Livonia, MI 48150
Phone: 888-432-5470
Website: www.tcns.org

Wound, Ostomy, and Continence Nurses Society
15000 Commerce Pkwy., Ste. C
Mt. Laurel, NJ 08054
Phone: 888-224-9626
Website: www.wocn.org

State and Territorial Nurses Associations

Alabama State Nurses Association
360 N. Hull St.
Montgomery, AL 36104-3658
Phone: 334-262-8321
Fax: 334-262-8578
Website: www.alabamanurses.org

Alaska Nurses Association
3701 E. Tudor Rd., Ste. 208
Anchorage, AK 99507-1069
Phone: 907-274-0827
Fax: 907-272-0292
Website: www.aknurse.org

Arizona Nurses Association
1850 E. Southern Ave., Ste. 1
Tempe, AZ 85282
Phone: 480-831-0404
Fax: 480-839-4780
Website: www.aznurse.org

Arkansas Nurses Association
1123 S. University Ave., #1015
Little Rock, AR 72204
Phone: 501-244-2363
Fax: 501-244-9903
Website: www.arna.org

ANA California
1121 L St., Ste. 409
Sacramento, CA 95814
Phone: 916-447-0225
Fax: 916-442-4394
Website: www.anacalifornia.org

Colorado Nurses Association
2170 S. Parker Rd., Ste. 145
Denver, CO 80231
Phone: 303-757-7483
Fax: 303-757-8833
Website: www.nurses-co.org

Connecticut Nurses Association
377 Research Pkwy., Ste. 2D
Meriden, CT 06450-7160
Phone: 203-238-1207
Fax: 203-238-3437
Website: www.ctnurses.org

Delaware Nurses Association
726 Loveville Rd., Ste. 3000
Hockessin, DE 19707
Phone: 302-239-3141
Fax: 302-998-3143
Website: www.denurses.org

IMPORTANT RESOURCES

District of Columbia Nurses Association
5100 Wisconsin Ave., NW, Ste. 306
Washington, DC 20016
Phone: 202-244-2705
Fax: 202-362-8285
Website: www.dcna.org

Florida Nurses Association
P.O. Box 536985
Orlando, FL 32853-6985
Phone: 407-896-3261
Fax: 407-896-9042
Website: www.floridanurse.org

Georgia Nurses Association
3032 Briarcliff Rd.
Atlanta, GA 30329-2655
Phone: 404-325-5536
Fax: 404-325-0407
Website: www.georgianurses.org

Guam Nurses Association
P.O. Box CG
Hagatna, Guam 96932
Phone: 671-787-4148
Fax: 671-477-6877

Hawaii Nurses Association
677 Ala Moana Blvd., Ste. 301
Honolulu, HI 96813
Phone: 808-531-1628
Fax: 808-524-2760
Website: www.hawaiinurses.org

Idaho Nurses Association
3525 Piedmont Rd. NE
Building Five, Ste. 300
Atlanta, GA 30305
Phone: 888-721-8904
FAX: 404-240-0998
Website: www.idahonurses.org

Illinois Nurses Association
105 W. Adams St., Ste. 2101
Chicago, IL 60603
Phone: 312-419-2900
Fax: 312-419-2920
Website: www.illinoisnurses.com

Indiana State Nurses Association
2915 N. High School Rd.
Indianapolis, IN 46224
Phone: 317-299-4575
Fax: 317-297-3525
Website: www.indiananurses.org

Iowa Nurses Association
2400 86th St. #32
Urbandale, IA 50322
Phone: 515-225-0495
Fax: 515-225-2201
Website: www.iowanurses.org

Kansas State Nurses Association
1109 SW Topeka Blvd.
Topeka, KS 66612-1602
Phone: 785-233-8638
Fax: 785-233-5222
Website: www.ksnurses.com

Kentucky Nurses Association
1400 S. First St.
P.O. Box 2616
Louisville, KY 40201-2616
Phone: 502-637-2546/800-348-5411
Fax: 502-637-8236
Website: www.kentucky-nurses.org

Louisiana State Nurses Association
5713 Superior Dr., Ste. A-6
Baton Rouge, LA 70816
Phone: 225-201-0993 or 800-457-6378
Fax: 225-201-0971
Website: www.lsna.org

ANA-Maine
P.O. Box 1205
Windham, ME 04062
Phone: 207-281-2091
Website: www.anamaine.org

Maryland Nurses Association
21 Governor's Court, Ste. 195
Baltimore, MD 21244
Phone: 410-944-5800
Fax: 410-944-5802
Website: www.marylandrn.org

Massachusetts Association of Registered Nurses
P.O. Box 285
Milton, MA 02186
Phone: 617-990-2856
Website: www.marnonline.org

Michigan Nurses Association
2310 Jolly Oak Rd.
Okemos, MI 48864-4599
Phone: 517-349-5640
Fax: 517-349-5818
Website: www.minurses.org

Minnesota Nurses Association
345 Randolph Ave. #200
St. Paul, MN 55102
Phone: 651-414-2800 or 800-536-4662
Fax: 651-695-7000
Website: www.mnnurses.org

Mississippi Nurses Association
31 Woodgreen Pl.
Madison, MS 39110
Phone: 601-898-0670
Fax: 601-898-0190
Website: www.msnurses.org

Missouri Nurses Association
1904 Bubba Ln.
P.O. Box 105228
Jefferson City, MO 65110-5228
Phone: 573-636-4623
Fax: 573-636-9576
Website: www.missourinurses.org

Montana Nurses Association
20 Old Montana State Hwy.
Montana City, MT 59634
Phone: 406-442-6710
Fax: 406-442-1841
Website: www.mtnurses.org

Nebraska Nurses Association
P.O. Box 82086
Lincoln, NE 68501-2086
Phone: 402-475-3859
Fax: 402-475-3961
Website: www.nebraskanurses.org

Nevada Nurses Association
P.O. Box 34660
Reno, NV 89533
Phone: 775-747-2333
Fax: 775-329-3334
Website: www.nvnurses.org

New Hampshire Nurses Association
210 N. State St., Ste. 1-A
Concord, NH 03301
Phone: 603-225-3783
Fax: 603-228-6672
Website: www.nhnurses.org

New Jersey State Nurses Association
1479 Pennington Rd.
Trenton, NJ 08618-2661
Phone: 609-883-5335
Fax: 609-883-5343
Website: www.njsna.org

New Mexico Nurses Association
P.O. Box 29658
Santa Fe, NM 87592-9658
Phone: 505-471-3324
Fax: 877-350-7499
Website: www.nmna.org

New York State Nurses Association
11 Cornell Rd.
Latham, NY 12110
Phone: 518-782-9400
Fax: 518-782-9530
Website: www.nysna.org

North Carolina Nurses Association
P.O. Box 12025
Raleigh, NC 27605
Phone: 919-821-4250/800-626-2153
Fax: 919-829-5807
Website: www.ncnurses.org

North Dakota Nurses Association
531 Airport Rd., Ste. D
Bismarck, ND 58504-6107
Phone: 701-223-1385
Fax: 701-223-0575
Website: www.ndna.org

Ohio Nurses Association
4000 E. Main St.
Columbus, OH 43213-2983
Phone: 614-237-5414
Fax: 614-237-6074
Website: www.ohnurses.org

Oklahoma Nurses Association
6414 N. Santa Fe, Ste. A
Oklahoma City, OK 73116
Phone: 405-840-3476
Fax: 405-840-3013
Website: www.oklahomanurses.org/

Oregon Nurses Association
18765 SW Boones Ferry Rd., Ste. 200
Tualatin, OR 97062
Phone: 503-293-0011
Fax: 503-293-0013
Website: www.oregonrn.org/

Pennsylvania State Nurses Association
2578 Interstate Dr., Ste. 101
Harrisburg, PA 17110-9601
Phone: 717-657-1222 or toll-free 888-707-7762
Fax: 717-657-3796
Website: www.panurses.org

Rhode Island State Nurses Association
150 Washington St., 4th Fl., Ste. 415
Providence, RI 02903
Phone: 401-331-5644
Fax: 401-331-5646
Website: www.risnarn.org

South Carolina Nurses Association
1821 Gadsden St.
Columbia, SC 29201
Phone: 803-252-4781
Fax: 803-779-3870
Website: www.scnurses.org

South Dakota Nurses Association
P.O. Box 1015
Pierre, SD 57501-1015
Phone: 605-945-4265
Fax: 888-425-3032
Website: www.sdnursesassociation.org

Tennessee Nurses Association
545 Mainstream Dr., Ste. 405
Nashville, TN 37228-1296
Phone: 615-254-0350
Fax: 615-254-0303
Website: www.tnaonline.org

Texas Nurses Association
7600 Burnet Rd., Ste. 440
Austin, TX 78757-1292
Phone: 512-452-0645/800-862-2022
Fax: 512-452-0648
Website: www.texasnurses.org

Utah Nurses Association
4505 S. Wasatch Blvd., Ste. 330B
Salt Lake City, UT 84124
Phone: 801-272-4510
Fax: 801-272-4322
Website: www.utahnursesassociation.com

Vermont State Nurses' Association
100 Dorset St., #13
South Burlington, VT 05403-6241
Phone: 802-651-8886
Fax: 802-651-8998
Website: www.vsna-inc.org

Virgin Islands State Nurses Association
P.O. Box 3617
Christiansted, US Virgin Islands 00822
Phone: 340-713-0293

Virginia Nurses Association
7113 Three Chopt Rd., Ste. 204
Richmond, VA 23226
Phone: 804-282-1808
Fax: 804-282-4916
Website: www.virginianurses.com

Washington State Nurses Association
575 Andover Park W., Ste. 101
Seattle, WA 98188-3321
Phone: 206-575-7979
Fax: 206-575-1908
Website: www.wsna.org

West Virginia Nurses Association
P.O. Box 1946
Charleston, WV 25327
Phone: 304-342-1169 or Toll Free: 800-400-1226
Fax: 304-414-3369
Website: www.wvnurses.org

Wisconsin Nurses Association
6117 Monona Dr. #1
Monona, WI 53716
Phone: 608-221-0383
Fax: 608-221-2788
Website: www.wisconsinnurses.org

Wyoming Nurses Association
2816 Dogwood Ave.
PMB 101
Gillette, WY 82716
Phone: 1-800-795-6381
Website: www.wyonurse.org

Placement Services and Job Searches

Many organizations nationwide provide employment services for healthcare workers. In fact, it is a growing field precisely because the number of jobs is growing so fast. The following list covers just a few of the organizations and government agencies nationwide working to identify available jobs in healthcare, link candidates to employers and vice versa, or aid in the actual hiring process.

If you have access to a computer, make the Internet part of your job-hunting process. Both private industry and government bureaus sponsor career- and employment-related websites such as www.careerbuilder.com and www.monster.com. We have also included some pertinent website listings here. You also can visit online forums and discussion groups that are frequented by healthcare professionals, where you can post your credentials, ask politely for referrals, or respond to specific job listings.

American Association of Managed Care Nurses, Inc. Job Placement Services
4435 Waterfront Dr., Ste. 101
Glen Allen, VA 23060
Phone: 804-527-9698
Fax: 804-747-5316
Website: www.aamcn.org

American Nursing Services
Phone: 800-444-NURS (6877)
Website: www.american-nurse.com

American Public Health Association CareerMart (online only)
Website: www.apha.org/career

CompHealth
4021 South 700 E., Ste. 300
Salt Lake City, UT 84107
Phone: 801-264-6400/800-453-3030
Fax: 801-264-6464
Website: www.comphealth.com

Department of Health and Human Services
200 Independence Ave. SW
Washington, DC 20201
Phone: 202-619-0257 / 877-696-6775
For 24-hour Job Information: 912-757-3000
Website: www.hhs.gov/jobs

Department of Veterans Affairs
810 Vermont Ave. NW
Washington, DC 20420
Phone: 202-273-5400
Website: www.va.gov

NurseWeek.com
Website: www.Nurseweek.com

NursingJobs.com
12400 High Bluff Dr.
San Diego, CA 92130
Phone: 877-435-2131
Website: www.nursingjobs.com

Nurse Web Search—The Nurse Directory
Website: www.nursewebsearch.com/nursing_employment.htm

NurseZone
12235 El Camino Real, Ste. 200
San Diego, CA 92130
Phone: 877-585-5010
Fax: 888-458-0197
Website: www.NurseZone.com

Homecare Organizations by State

One of your best bets in finding a job is one of the more than 80,000 home-healthcare providers operating in the United States as of 2009. The National Association for Home Care (NAHC) defines homecare organizations as home-health agencies, homecare-aide organizations, and hospices. Types of homecare agencies include visiting-urse associations (VNAs), public government-agencies, proprietary for-profit agencies, private not-for-profit agencies, and hospital-based agencies.

Members of the NAHC are featured in the following state-by-state listing of homecare organizations.

NATIONAL
Gentiva Home Health & Hospice
Corporate Office
Gentiva Health Services, Inc.
3350 Riverwood Pkwy., Ste. 1400
Atlanta, GA 30339
Phone: 770-951-6450
Website: www.gentiva.com

Kaiser Permanente
Website: www.kaiserpermanente.org

ALABAMA
Home Care Association of Alabama
P.O. Box 3238
Montgomery, AL 36109
Phone: 205-991-0081
Fax: 205-278-5822
Website: www.homecarealabama.org

Lanier Home Health Services
1806 44th St.
Valley, AL 36854
Phone: 334-756-1950
Fax: 334-756-1970
E-mail: dveal@lanierhospital.com

ALASKA
Alaska Home Care & Hospice Association
3701 East Tudor Rd., Ste. 208
Anchorage, AK 99507
Phone: 907-274-1066

ARIZONA
Arizona Association for Home Care
3933 S. McClintock Dr., Ste. 505
Tempe, AZ 85282
Phone: 480-491-0540
Fax: 480-603-4141
Website: www.azhomecare.org

ARKANSAS
Arkansas Hospital Association
419 Natural Resources Dr.
Little Rock, AK 72205-1576
Phone: 501-224-7878
Fax: 501-224-0519
Website: www.arkhospitals.org

Home Care Association of Arkansas
411 South Victory, Ste. 205
Little Rock, AK 72201
Phone: 501-376-2273
Fax: 501-376-7107
Website: www.homecareassociationarkansas.org

Home Health Professionals
P.O. Box 704
Blytheville, AK 72316
Phone: 870-762-1825
Fax: 870-762-2299

CALIFORNIA
Area Administrator, San Diego Home Health & Hospice
Kaiser Foundation Hospital Home Health
10992 San Diego Mission Rd. 3rd Fl.
San Diego, CA 92108
Phone: 619-641-4663
Fax: 619-641-4110

California Association for Health Services at Home
3780 Rosin Ct., Ste. 190
Sacramento, CA 95834
Phone: 916-641-5795
Fax: 916-641-5881
Website: www.cahsah.org

COLORADO
Home Care Association of Colorado
7853 East Arapahoe Rd., Ste. 2100
Englewood, CO 80112
Phone: 303-694-4728
Fax: 303-694-4869
Website: www.hcaconline.org

Northwest Colorado VNA/HQ
940 Central Park Dr., Ste. 101
Steamboat Springs, CO 80487
Phone: 970/-879-1632
Fax: 970-870-1326

CONNECTICUT
Connecticut Association for Home Care, Inc.
110 Barnes Rd.
P.O. Box 90
Wallingford, CT 06492-0090
Phone: 203-265-9931
Fax: 203-949-0031
Website: www.cthomecare.org

New England Home Health Care (NEHHC)
28 Gilman Plaza
Bangor, ME 04401
Phone: 207-945-3374
Toll-free: 1-800-287-0338
Fax: 207-942-1022

DELAWARE
Delaware Association of Home and Community Care
DAHCC
c/o P.O. Box 7603
Wilmington, DE 19803
Website: http://dahcc.org

St. Francis Hospital Home Health Care Program
Seventh and Clayton Sts.
Wilmington, DE 19805
Phone: 302-575-8420
Website: www.stfrancishealthcare.org

Delaware Hospice Association
800/838-9800
Website: www.delawarehospice.org
Dover Office
911 South DuPont Highway
Dover, DE 19901
Phone: 302-678-4444
Fax: 302-678-4451

Milford Office
Delaware Hospice Center
100 Patriots Way
Milford, DE 19963
Phone: 302-856-7717
Fax: 302-422-7315

Wilmington Office
3515 Silverside Rd.
Wilmington, DE 19810
Phone: 302-478-5707
Fax: 302-479-2597

FLORIDA
Associated Home Health (Dade County) #1
FL LIC—HHA219830961
5790 NW 72nd Ave.
Miami, FL 33166
Tel: 305-917-0363
Fax: 305-917-0368

Associated Home Health (Broward County) #2
FL LIC—HHA299991811
3313 W. Commercial Blvd., Ste. 114
Fort Lauderdale, FL 33309
Phone: 954-938-3500
Fax: 954-938-3509

Associated Home Health (Palm Beach County) #3
FL LIC—HHA299991773
1710 Corporate Dr.
Boynton Beach, FL 33426
Phone: 561-272-9494
Fax: 561-276-5580

Associated Home Health (St. Lucie County) #4
FL LIC—HHA299991834
1401 S.E. Goldtree Dr., Ste. 101
Port St. Lucie, FL 34952
Phone: 772-337-3600
Fax: 772-337-4662

Associated Home Health (Indian River County) #5
FL LIC—HHA 299992033
7400 US Hwy. #1
Vero Beach, FL 32967
Phone: 772-770-1100
Fax: 772-770-9164

Associated Home Health (Tampa/Hillsborough County) #6
FL LIC—HHA29991170
4714 N. Armenia Ave., Ste. 101
Tampa, FL 33603
Phone: 813-962-0070
Fax: 813-908-1448

Associated Home Health (Brevard County) #7
FL LIC—HHA299991743
3200 N. Wickham Rd., Ste. 4
Melbourne, FL 32935
Phone: 321-242-8228
Fax: 321-242-8401

Associated Home Health (Clearwater/Pinellas County) #8
FL LIC—HHA299991742
2370 Drew St., Ste. A, Unit 1, Building 1
Clearwater, FL 33765
Phone: 727-726-7400
Fax: 727-726-7474

Associated Home Health (New Port Richie/ Pasco County) #9
FL LIC—HHA299991875
5833 US Hwy. 19, Ste. 12
New Port Richey, FL 34652
Phone: 727-841-8199
Fax: 727-841-8950

Associated Home Health (Lakeland/ Polk County) #10
FL LIC—HHA299992338
316 East Pine St.
Lakeland, FL 33801
Phone: 863-682-8538 / 863-682-8768
Fax: 863-688-3451

GEORGIA
Georgia Association for Home Health Agencies, Inc.
2100 Roswell Rd.
Ste. 200C—PMB 1107
Marietta, GA 30062
Phone: 770-565-4531
Fax: 770-565-1739
Website: www.gahha.org

Georgia Association of Community Care Providers
P.O. Box 3364
Gainesville, GA 30503
Phone: 678-943-2617
Fax: 678-262-9951
Website: www.gaccp.org

HAWAII
Healthcare Association of Hawaii
932 Ward Ave., Ste. 430
Honolulu, HI 96814-2126
Phone: 808-521-8961
Fax: 808-599-2879
Website: www.hah.org

CareResource Hawaii
Website: www.careresourcehawaii.org
Oahu—Main Office:
680 Iwilei Rd., Ste. 660
Honolulu , HI 96817
Tel: 808-599-4999
Fax: 808-599-8880

Hilo Branch Office
100 Pauahi St., Ste. 214
Hilo, HI 96720
Phone: 808-935-2718

Kona Branch Office
75-167 Kalani St., Ste. #206
Kailua-Kona, HI 96740
Phone: 808-326-7021

Maui Branch Office
355 Hukilike St., Ste. 126
Kahului, HI 96732
Phone: 808-871-2115

Molokai Branch Office
10 N. Mohala St., Ste. 201
Kaunakakai, HI 96748
Phone: 808-553-9851

IDAHO

Idaho Home Health & Hospice
826 Eastland Dr.
Twin Falls, ID 83301
Phone: 208-734-4061
Fax: 208-733-5980

Oneida County Hospital Home Care
150 N. 200 W.
Malad City, ID 83252
Phone: 208-766-5805
Fax: 208-766-4819

Panhandle Health District Home Health Division
8500 North Atlas Rd.
Hayden, ID 83835
Phone: 208-415-5160
Fax: 208-415-5161

ILLINOIS

Addus HealthCare
2401 S. Plum Grove Rd.
Palatine, IL 60067
Phone: 877-233-8744
Fax: 847-303-5376

All Help Health Services, Inc.
6160 N. Cicero Ave., Ste. 303
Chicago, IL 60646
Phone: 773-355-5417
Fax: 773-283-9320

Palos Community Hospital Home Health Care and Hospice
15295 East 127th St.
Lemont, IL 60439-7405
Phone: 630-257-1111
Fax: 630-257-1461

Riverside Home Health Care
1905 West Court St., Entrance D
Kankakee, IL 60901
Phone: 815-935-3272
Fax: 815-937-7961

INDIANA

Hoosier Uplands Home Health and Hospice
500 W. Main St.
Mitchell, IN 47446
Phone: 812-849-4447
Fax: 812-849-3068
Website: www.hoosieruplands.org

Indiana Association for Home & Hospice Care, LLC
6320-G Rucker Rd.
Indianapolis, IN 46220
Phone: 317) 775-6675
Fax: 317) 775-6674
Website: www.ind-homecare.org

Regional Home Health Care, Inc.
525 West Bristol St., Ste. A
P.O. Box 128
Elkhart, IN 46515-0128
Phone: 574-295-1111
Fax: 574-295-4444

St. Margaret Mercy Healthcare Centers
5454 Hohman Ave.
Hammond, IN 46320-1931
Phone: 219-933-2074
Fax: 219-933-2585
Website: http://franciscanstmargaret.org

IOWA

Advanced Home Health Care, Ltd
1525 Mount Pleasant St.
Burlington, IA 52601
Phone: 319-753-6270
Fax: 319-753-6237

Finley Home Healthcare
1333 Delhi St.
Dubuque, IA 52001
Phone: 563-589-2553
Fax: 563-557-2864

Heartland Hospice Services—Davenport
4340 East 53rd St.
Davenport, IA 52807
Phone: 563-359-3540
Fax: 563-359-9092

Iowa Health Care Association
Iowa Center for Assisted Living
1775 90th St.
West Des Moines, IA 50266-7726
Phone: 515.978.2204 or 800.422.3106
Fax: 515.978.2209
Website: www.iowahealthcare.org

Iowa Health Home Care Hospice
11333 Aurora Ave.
Urbandale, IA 50322
Phone: 515-557-3287
Fax: 515-557-3290

KANSAS
Carondelet Home Care Services
11050 Roe Ave., Ste. 120
Overland Park, KS 66211
Phone: 913-529-4800
Fax: 913-345-9129

Community Home Health
100 W. 8th
Onaga, KS 66521
Phone: 785-889-7200
Fax: 785/889-4808

Kansas Home Care Association KHCA
2738 SW Santa Fe Dr.
Topeka, KS 66614
Phone: 785-478-3640
Fax: 785-286-1835
Website: www.kshomecare.org

Shawnee Mission Home Health Care
7312 Antioch Rd.
Shawnee Mission, KS 66204
Phone: 913-676-2163
Fax: 913-676-2363

KENTUCKY
Caldwell County Hospital Home Health Agency
1310 Hwy. 62 West
P.O. Box 410
Princeton, KY 42445
Phone: 270-365-2011
Fax: 270-365-9433

Lourdes HomeCare/Hospice
2855 Jackson St., Ste. 5
Paducah, KY 42003
Phone: 270-415-3600
Fax: 270-444-2379

Methodist Hospital HomeCare
110 Second St.
Henderson, KY 42420
Phone: 270-869-1997
Fax: 270-869-1884

The Visiting Nurse Association of Greater Cincinnati and Northern Kentucky
2400 Reading Rd.
Cincinnati, Ohio 45202
Phone: 513-345-8000
Phone: 800-345-8085
Website: www.thevna.org

LOUISIANA
Complete Home Health, Inc.
1753 Bertrand Dr.
Lafayette, LA 70508
Phone: 337-233-0079
Fax: 337-233-7414

HomeCare Association of Louisiana
850 Kaliste Saloom Rd., Ste. 123
Lafayette, LA 70508
Toll Free: 1-800-283-HCLA
Phone: 337-231-0080
Fax: 337-231-0089
Website: www.hclanet.org

MAINE
Home Care Alliance of Maine
20 Middle St.
Augusta, ME 04330
Phone: 207-623-0345
Fax: 207-623-7141
Website: www.homecarealliance.org

SMMC Visiting Nurses
72 Main St.
Kennebunk, ME 04043-0739
Phone: 207-985-1000 or 800-794-3546
Fax: 207-985-6715

MARYLAND/DISTRICT OF COLUMBIA
Chesapeake-Potomac Home Health Agency, Inc.
7627 Leonardtown Rd.
Leonardtown, MD 20637
Phone: 301-274-9000
Fax: 301-274-9009
Website: http://cphha.org

Maryland National Capital Homecare Association
6919 Baltimore National Pike, Ste. F
Frederick, MD 21702
Phone: 301-473-9801
Fax: 301-473-9803

MASSACHUSETTS
**Home & Health Care Association
of Massachusetts**
31 James Ave., Ste. 780
Boston, MA 02116
Phone: 617-482-8830
Fax: 617-426-0509
Website: www.hhcam.org

**Massachusetts Council for Home Care
Aide Services**
174 Portland St., 5th Fl.
Boston, MA 02114
Phone: 617-224-4141
Fax: 617-227-1190
Website: http://mahomecareaides.com

VNA of Greater Lowell
336 Central St.
Lowell, MA 01852
Phone: 978-459-9343
Toll-free: 800-349-8585
Fax: 978-441-0007
Website: www.vnalowell.org

MICHIGAN
Michigan Home Health Association
2140 University Park Dr., Ste. 220
Okemos, MI 48864
Phone: 517-349-8089
Fax: 517-349-8090
Website: www.mhha.org

Porter Hills Home Health
4450 Cascade Rd., Ste. 300
Grand Rapids, MI 49546
Phone: 616-949-5140
Fax: 616-954-1795
Website: www.porterhills.org/Homecare.asp

Quality Home Health Care Services of Michigan
23800 W. 10 Mile Rd., Ste. 250
Southfield, MI 48033
Phone: 248-350-0014
Fax: 248-350-3298
Website: www.qualityhomehealthcare.net

MINNESOTA
Minnesota HomeCare Association
1711 West County Rd. B, Ste. 211S
St. Paul, MN 55113-4036
Phone: 651-635-0607
Fax: 651-635-0043
Website: www.mnhomecare.org

Fairview Home Care and Hospice
2450—26th Ave. S.
Minneapolis, MN 55406
Phone: 612-721-2491
Fax: 612-728-2400
Website: www.fairview.org/homecare

MISSISSIPPI
Kare-In-Home Health Services
Website: http://kareinhome.com
Gulfport, MS
10281 Corporate Dr.
Gulfport, MS 39503
Phone: 228-604-2155
Phone: 800-898-0953

Lucedale, MS
53 Dewey St.
Lucedale, MS 39452
Phone: 601-766-3429
Phone: 800-485-1329

Pascagoula, MS
4509 Hospital St.
Pascagoula, MS 39581
Phone: 228-762-9999
Phone: 877-567-2559

Picayune, MS
4201 US Hwy 11 N, Ste. B
Picayune, MS 39466
Phone: 601-799-2088
Phone: 866-757-5273

Mississippi Association for Home Care
134 Fairmont St., Ste. B
Clinton, MS 39056
Phone: 601-924-2275
Fax: 601-924-0720
Website: www.mahc.org

MISSOURI
Carondelet Home Care Services
809 NE Anderson Ln.
Lees Summit, MO 64064
Phone: 816-655-5494
Fax: 816-655-5496
Website: www.carondelethealth.org

John Knox Village Home Health
400 Northwest Murray Rd.
Lee's Summit, MO 64081
Phone Toll Free: 1-800-892-5669
Phone Local: (816) 251-8000
Fax: 816) 246-4739
Website: http://jkv.org

Missouri Alliance for Home Care
2420 Hyde Park Rd., Ste. A
Jefferson City, MO 65109
Phone: 573-634-7772
Fax: 573-634-4374
Website: www.homecaremissouri.org

St. John's Home Care—Mountain View
Aurora: 417-678-2158 or 866-293-1507
Lebanon: 417-588-5900 or 877-500-9500
Mountain View: 417-934-2347 or 800-633-0071
Shell Knob: 417-858-2933 or 800-730-8469
Springfield: 417-820-4374 or 800-595-7167
Website: www.stjohns.com/homecarehospice

MONTANA
Montana Hospital Association: An Association of Montana Health Care Providers
P.O. Box 5119
Helena, MT 59604
Phone: 406-442-1911
Fax: 406-443-3894
Website: www.mtha.org

Marcus Daley Home Care and Hospice
1200 Westwood Dr.
Hamilton, MT 59840
Phone: 406-363-6503
Fax: 406-363-2866

NEBRASKA
Nebraska Association of Home and Community Health Agencies
1633 Normandy Ct., Ste. A
Lincoln, NE 68512
Phone: 402-423-0718
Fax: 402-476-6547
Website: www.nebraskahomecare.org

Saint Francis Medical Center Home Care Services
2116 W. Faidley Ave.
Grand Island, NE 68802
Phone: 308-398-5470
Fax: 308-398-5363

NEVADA
Nevada Health Care Association
35 E. Horizon Ridge Pkwy., #110-137
Henderson, NV 89002
Phone: 866-307-0942
Website: www.nvhca.org

Saint Rose Dominican Hospital Home Health Services
1125 American Pacific Dr., Ste. E
Henderson, NV 89074
Phone: 702-616-6555
Fax: 702-566-9157
Website: www.strosehospitals.org

NEW HAMPSHIRE
Home Care Association of New Hampshire
8 Green St.
Concord, NH 03301
Phone: 603-225-5597
Fax: 603-225-5817
Website: www.homecarenh.org

Rockingham VNA & Hospice
137 Epping Rd.
Exeter, NH 03079
Phone: 603-893-2900
Fax: 603-382-6246

NEW JERSEY
The Home Care Association of New Jersey
485D Route 1 S., Ste. 210
Iselin, NJ 08830
Phone: 732-877-1100 or 609-275-6100
Fax: 732-877-1101 or 609-936-9349
Website: www.homecarenj.org

New Jersey Hospital Association
760 Alexander Rd.
P.O. Box 1
Princeton, NJ 08543-0001
Phone: 609-275-4000
Fax: 609-275-4265 fax
Website: www.njha.com

VNA of Central Jersey, Inc.
Woodbridge Regional Office
91 Main St.
Woodbridge, NJ 07095
Phone: 732-634-6110
Website: www.vnacj.org

NEW MEXICO
Lovelace Sandia Home Care
5403 Gibson SE
Albuquerque, NM 87108
Phone: 505-872-6511
Fax: 505-872-6547

New Mexico Association for Home and Hospice Care
3200 Carlisle Blvd., NE, Ste. 117
Albuquerque, NM 87110
Phone: 505-889-4556
Fax: 505-889-4928
Website: www.nmahc.org

NEW YORK
Health Care Association of New York State
One Empire Dr.
Rensselaer, NY 12144
Phone: 518-431-7600
Fax: 518/431-7915
Website: www.hanys.org

Home Care Association of New York State, Inc.
194 Washington Ave., Ste. 400
Albany, NY 12210
Phone: 518-426-8764
Fax: 518-426-8788
Website: www.hcanys.org

New York State Association of Health Care Providers, Inc.
99 Troy Rd., Ste. 200
East Greenbush, NY 12061
Phone: 518-463-1118
Fax: 518-463-1606
Website: www.nyshcp.org

VNA of Hudson Valley, Inc.
540 White Plains Rd., Ste. 300
Tarrytown, NY 10591-5132
Phone: 914-666-7616
Website: http://vnahv.com

NORTH CAROLINA
Association for Home Care and Hospice of North Carolina, Inc.
3101 Industrial Dr.
Raleigh, NC 27609
Phone: 919-848-3450
Fax: 919-848-2355
Website: www.homeandhospicecare.org

Carolinas Center for Hospice and End of Life Care
North Carolina Office
1230 SE Maynard Rd., Ste. 203
Cary, NC 27511
Phone: 919-459-5380
Toll-free: 800-662-8859
Website: www.cchospice.org

Piedmont Home Care
2160 B Country Club Rd.
Winston Salem, NC 27104
Phone: 336-724-1197
Website: http://piedmonthomehealth.com

NORTH DAKOTA
Jamestown Regional Medical Center
Home Health/Hospice
2422 20th St.
Jamestown, ND 58401
Phone: 701-952-4847
Website: www.jamestownhospital.com

North Dakota Association for Home Care
P.O. Box 2175
Bismarck, ND 58502-2175
Phone: 701-224-1815
Fax: 701-224-9824
Website: www.aptnd.com/ndahc

OHIO
Associated Home Health
215 Main St.
Wintersville, OH 43953
Phone: 740-264-6311
Fax: 740-264-6120

Hospice of the Western Reserve
17876 St. Clair Ave.
Cleveland, OH 44110-2602
Phone: 800-707-8922
Website: www.hospicewr.org

Ohio Council for Home Care
2800 Corporate Exchange Dr., Ste. 225
Columbus, OH 43231
Phone: 614-885-0434
Fax: 614-899-0192
Website: www.homecareohio.org

Ohio Hospice & Palliative Care Organization
855 South Wall St.
Columbus, OH 43206
Phone: 614-763-0036
Toll Free: 1-800-776-9513
Fax: 614-763-0050
Website: www.ohpco.org

OKLAHOMA
Choice Home Health & Choice Hospice
1 NW 64th St., #A
Oklahoma City, OK 73116-9105
Phone: 405-879-3470
Fax: 405-879-1625

Oklahoma Association for Home Care
8108 NW Tenth, Ste. C3
Oklahoma City, OK 73127
Phone: 405-495-5995
Fax: 405-495-5993
Website: www.oahc.com

OREGON
Grande Ronde Hospital Home Care and Hospice Services
P.O. Box 3290
La Grande, OR 97850
Phone: 541-963-1453
Fax: 541-963-1872
Website: www.grh.org/srvHome.aspx

Oregon Association for Home Care
4676 Commercial St. SE #449
Salem, OR 97302
Phone: 503-364-2733 or 800-352-7230
Fax: 877-458-8348
Website: www.oahc.org

PENNSYLVANIA
Abington Health Center—Schilling Campus
2510 Maryland Rd., Ste. 250
Willow Grove, PA 19090-0520
Phone: 215-481-5800
Fax: 215-481-5850
Website: www.amh.org/services/home-care

Pennsylvania Homecare Association
20 Erford Rd., Ste. 115
Lemoyne, PA 17043
Phone: 717-975-9448
Fax: 717-975-9456
Website: www.pahomecare.org

RHODE ISLAND
Rhode Island Partnership for Home Care, Inc.
57 Kilvert St., Ste. 101
Warwick, RI 02886
Phone: 401-732-1010
Fax: 401-732-1010
Website: www.riphc.org

VNA Rhode Island
475 Kilvert St.
Warwick, RI 02886
Phone: 401-574-4900
Toll free: 800-638-6274
Website: www.vnari.org

VNS and Hospice of Newport and Bristol Counties
1184 East Main Rd.
P.O. Box 690
Portsmouth, RI 02871
Phone: 401-682-2100
Fax: 401-682-2887
Website: www.vnsri.com

SOUTH CAROLINA
Carolinas Center for Hospice and End of Life Care
South Carolina Office
1350 Browning Rd.
Columbia, SC 29210
Phone: 803-791-4220
Website: www.cchospice.org

SOUTH DAKOTA
Avera Scared Heart Health Care Services
501 Summit
Yankton, SD 57078
Phone: 605-668-8000
Website: www.avera.org/sacred-heart/index.aspx

South Dakota Association of Healthcare Organizations
3708 Brooks Pl.
Sioux Falls, SD 57106
Phone: 605-361-2281
Fax: 605-361-5175
Website: www.sdaho.org

TENNESSEE
Tennessee Association for Home Care, Inc.
131 Donelson Pike
Nashville, Tennessee 37214-2901
Phone: 615-885-3399
Fax: 615-885-4191
Website: www.tahc-net.org

UT Medical Center Home Health
The University of Tennessee Medical Center
1924 Alcoa Hwy., Knoxville, TN 37920
Phone: 865-305-9000
Website: www.utmedicalcenter.org/departments/patient
-services/home-care-services

TEXAS
Home Health Care of North Central Texas, Inc.
P.O. Box 1298
1116 Halsell St., Ste. 300
Bridgeport, TX 76426
Phone: 940-683-3300
Fax: 940-683-3302
Website: www.homehealthoftexas.com

Texas Association for Home Care
3737 Executive Center Dr., Ste. 268
Austin, TX 78731
Phone: 512-338-9293
Fax: 512-338-9496
Website: www.tahc.org

UTAH
Applegate HomeCare & Hospice
Website: www.applegatehospice.com/Pages/Home.aspx
　Main Office, Ogden: 801-621-6950
　American Fork Office: (801-763-0101
　Bountiful Office: (801-296-2245
　Coeur d'Alene Office: (208-765-2273
　Heber Office: 435-654-5983
　Layton Office: 801-614-0052
　Ogden Office: 801-394-3250
　Park City Office: 435-647-3765
　Salt Lake Office: 801-261-3023
　St. George Office: 435-628-1569

Utah Association for Home Care
1327 South 900 East
Salt Lake City, UT 84105
Phone: 801-466-7210
Website: www.ua4hc.org

VERMONT
Franklin County Home Health Agency, Inc.
3 Home Health Circle, Ste. 1
Saint Albans, VT 05478
Phone: 802-527-7531
Fax: 802-527-7533
Website: www.fchha.org

Rutland Area VNA and Hospice
P.O. Box 787
Rutland, VT
Phone: 802-775-0568
Website: www.ravnah.org

VIRGINIA
Virginia Association for Home Care
8001 Franklin Farms Dr., Ste. 110
Richmond, Virginia 23229
Phone: 804-285-8636
Phone: 800-755-8636
Fax: 804-288-3303
Website: www.vahc.org

Virginia Hospital and Health Care Association
4200 Innslake Dr., Ste. 203
Glen Allen, VA 23060
Phone: 804-965-1227
Website: www.vhha.com

WASHINGTON
Group Health Cooperative Home & Community Services
P.O. Box 34590
Seattle, WA 98124-1590
Phone: 1-888-901-4636
Website: www.ghc.org

Home Care Association of Washington
P.O. Box 2016
Edmonds, WA 98020
Phone: 425-775-8120
Fax: 425-771-9588
Website: www.hcaw.org

WEST VIRGINIA
Panhandle Home Health
208 Old Mill Rd.
Martinsburg, WV 25401
Phone Local: 304-263-5680
Phone Toll Free: 1-800-397-7444
Fax: 304-267-1532
Website: http://panhandlehomehealth.org

West Virginia Council of Home Care Agencies, Inc.
Route 1 Box 190
Elk Fork Rd.
Middlebourne WV 26149
Phone: 304-758-4312
Website: www.wvhomecareassociation.com

WISCONSIN
Wisconsin Homecare Organization
2937 Maple View Dr.
Madison, WI 53719
Phone: 608-212-1981
Fax: 608-271-6351
Website: www.wishomecare.org

WYOMING
Central Wyoming Hospice Program
319 South Wilson St.
Casper, WY 82601
Phone: 307-577-4832
Fax: 307-577-4841
Website: www.cwhp.org

Cheyenne Regional Medical Center Home Care Services
214 East 23rd St.
Cheyenne, WY 82001
Phone: 307-633-7000
Fax: 307-633-7075
Website: www.crmcwy.org

Directories

Consult the directories on the following list for . . . well, mostly more lists. Just like your local phone book, these directories offer you long lists of names, addresses, phone numbers, and contact persons—in this case, at hospitals, HMOs, private practices, geriatric facilities, and more. Directories can be especially useful when you're researching education programs or scoping out job prospects in your region or across the country.

AHA Guide to the Health Care Field
American Hospital Association
One N. Franklin, 27th Floor
Chicago, IL 60606
Toll Free: 800-242-2626
Website: www.ahaonlinestore.com
(hospitals, clinics, other healthcare organizations)

American Association of Homes and Services for the Aging
2519 Connecticut Ave., NW
Washington, DC 20008-1520
Toll-Free: 800-508-9442
Phone: 770-442-8633, ext 369
Website: www.aahsa.org/public/books.htm
(assorted books on geriatric care)

American Hospital Directory
3630-A Brownsboro Rd., #200
Louisville, KY 40207-1861
Email: inbox@ahd.com
Fax: 502-899-7738
Website: www.ahd.com
(hospitals)

American Medical Group Association
1422 Duke St.
Alexandria, VA 22314-3430
Phone: 703-838-0033
Fax: 703-548-1890
Website: www.amga.org
(assorted books on physicians-private medical practices)

Assisted Living and Extended Care Facilities Hospital Blue Book
Managed Healthcare Organizations
Billian's HealthDATA Group
2100 Powers Ferry Rd.
Atlanta, GA 30339
Phone:770-955-8484
Fax: 770-955-8485
Website: www.billianshealthdata.com
(assorted directories on healthcare facilities, hospitals, and managed care organizations)

Case Management Resource Guide
AAHP/Dorland Directory of Health Plans
Directory of Physician Groups & Networks
Dorland Healthcare Information
1500 Walnut St., Ste. 1000
Philadelphia, PA 19102
Phone: 215-875-1212
Toll-Free: 800-784-2332
Fax: 215-735-3966
Product Inquiries: info@dorlandhealth.com
Website: www.dorlandhealth.com
(health care facilities, HMOs, adult day care, cancer centers, other)

Directory of Privately Owned Hospitals, Hospital Management Companies and Health Systems, Residential Treatment Facilities and Centers, and Key Management Personnel
Federation of American Hospitals
1405 N. Pierce, Ste. 311
Little Rock, AR 72207
Phone: 501-661-9555
(health care facilities nationwide)

Medical and Health Information Directory
Gale Research Company
P.O. Box 9187
Farmington Hills, MI 48333-9187
Phone: 800-877-GALE
Fax: 800-414-5043
Website: www.galegroup.com
E-mail: galeord@gale.com
(medical associations, schools, federal agencies, other)

APPENDIX: NURSING ASSISTANT/ NURSE AIDE PRACTICE EXAM QUESTION OUTLINE

You can use the charts on the pages that follow to assess the areas in which you need more study. The column on the left indicates the topics tested, and the right column indicates the question numbers in that topic.

Nursing Assistant/Nurse Aide Practice Exam 1

PHYSICAL CARE SKILLS	
TOPIC	**QUESTION NUMBERS**
Activities of Daily Living ■ Hygiene ■ Dressing and Grooming ■ Nutrition and Hydration ■ Elimination ■ Rest/Sleep/Comfort	2, 5, 8, 10, 17, 31, 52, 54, 68, 69
Basic Nursing Skills ■ Infection Control ■ Safety/Emergency ■ Therapeutic/Technical Procedures ■ Data Collection and Reporting	3, 4, 6, 7, 11, 15, 16, 21, 24, 25, 26 27, 30, 32, 33, 34, 35, 36, 37, 38, 39 40, 41, 42, 43, 45, 47, 61, 62, 65, 66
Restorative Skills ■ Prevention ■ Self-Care/Independence	1, 18, 19

PSYCHOSOCIAL CARE SKILLS	
TOPIC	**QUESTION NUMBERS**
Emotional and Mental Health Needs	9, 47, 49, 51, 53, 55, 56, 70
Spiritual and Cultural Needs	57, 58

ROLE OF THE NURSE AIDE	
TOPIC	**QUESTION NUMBERS**
Communication	12, 13, 20, 23, 59, 64
Client Rights	28, 29, 46, 48, 50
Legal and Ethical Behavior	45, 60, 67
Member of the Healthcare Team	14, 22, 44, 63

Nursing Assistant/Nurse Aide Practice Exam 2

PHYSICAL CARE SKILLS	
TOPIC	**QUESTION NUMBERS**
Activities of Daily Living ■ Hygiene ■ Dressing and Grooming ■ Nutrition and Hydration ■ Elimination ■ Rest/Sleep/Comfort	8, 28, 29, 30, 33, 35, 60
Basic Nursing Skills ■ Infection Control ■ Safety/Emergency ■ Therapeutic/Technical Procedures ■ Data Collection and Reporting	1, 4, 5, 7, 9, 10, 11, 12, 13, 16, 17 18, 19, 20, 21, 22, 23, 24, 25, 27, 31 34, 36, 37, 38, 50, 56, 59, 64, 66
Restorative Skills ■ Prevention ■ Self-Care/Independence	2, 3, 6, 14, 15, 32, 49

PSYCHOSOCIAL CARE SKILLS	
TOPIC	**QUESTION NUMBERS**
Emotional and Mental Health Needs	41, 42, 43, 46
Spiritual and Cultural Needs	39, 65

ROLE OF THE NURSE AIDE	
TOPIC	**QUESTION NUMBERS**
Communication	26, 44, 57, 58, 59, 68
Client Rights	40, 45, 51, 52, 53, 54, 55, 67, 69
Legal and Ethical Behavior	47, 48, 61, 70
Member of the Healthcare Team	62, 63

Nursing Assistant/Nurse Aide Practice Exam 3

PHYSICAL CARE SKILLS	
TOPIC	**QUESTION NUMBERS**
Activities of Daily Living ■ Hygiene ■ Dressing and Grooming ■ Nutrition and Hydration ■ Elimination ■ Rest/Sleep/Comfort	13, 16, 24, 35, 37, 39, 53, 70
Basic Nursing Skills ■ Infection Control ■ Safety/Emergency ■ Therapeutic/Technical Procedures ■ Data Collection and Reporting	2, 3, 4, 5, 6, 10, 11, 12, 14, 15 17, 18, 20, 22, 23, 25, 26, 27, 28 29, 30, 31, 32, 33, 34, 38, 42, 47, 48, 57
Restorative Skills ■ Prevention ■ Self-Care/Independence	1, 8, 56

PSYCHOSOCIAL CARE SKILLS	
TOPIC	**QUESTION NUMBERS**
Emotional and Mental Health Needs	7, 59, 60, 61, 63, 64
Spiritual and Cultural Needs	58, 65

ROLE OF THE NURSE AIDE	
TOPIC	**QUESTION NUMBERS**
Communication	46, 49, 52, 62
Client Rights	21, 44, 45, 54, 55, 69
Legal and Ethical Behavior	19, 40, 41, 43, 50
Member of the Healthcare Team	36, 51, 66, 67, 68

Nursing Assistant/Nurse Aide Practice Exam 4

PHYSICAL CARE SKILLS	
TOPIC	**QUESTION NUMBERS**
Activities of Daily Living	4, 33, 34, 35, 36, 61
■ Hygiene	
■ Dressing and Grooming	
■ Nutrition and Hydration	
■ Elimination	
■ Rest/Sleep/Comfort	
Basic Nursing Skills	1, 2, 5, 8, 11, 12, 13, 14, 15, 17, 18
■ Infection Control	19, 20, 21, 22, 23, 24, 25, 26, 27, 28
■ Safety/Emergency	29, 30, 31, 32, 38, 57
■ Therapeutic/Technical Procedures	
■ Data Collection and Reporting	
Restorative Skills	3, 7, 9, 10, 37, 39
■ Prevention	
■ Self-Care/Independence	

PSYCHOSOCIAL CARE SKILLS	
TOPIC	**QUESTION NUMBERS**
Emotional and Mental Health Needs	40, 41, 42, 43, 44, 45, 46, 48, 58
Spiritual and Cultural Needs	47

ROLE OF THE NURSE AIDE	
TOPIC	**QUESTION NUMBERS**
Communication	49, 50, 51, 52, 54
Client Rights	53, 60, 62, 64, 66
Legal and Ethical Behavior	55, 56, 63, 65
Member of the Healthcare Team	6, 16, 59, 67, 68, 69, 70

Nursing Assistant/Nurse Aide Practice Exam 5

PHYSICAL CARE SKILLS	
TOPIC	**QUESTION NUMBERS**
Activities of Daily Living ■ Hygiene ■ Dressing and Grooming ■ Nutrition and Hydration ■ Elimination ■ Rest/Sleep/Comfort	2, 3, 5, 10, 14, 20, 21, 23
Basic Nursing Skills ■ Infection Control ■ Safety/Emergency ■ Therapeutic/Technical Procedures ■ Data Collection and Reporting	1, 4, 6, 7, 8, 11, 12, 13, 15, 17, 18, 22, 25 26, 27, 28, 29, 32, 33, 34, 35, 37, 38, 39 41, 42, 43, 44, 45, 46, 52, 60
Restorative Skills ■ Prevention ■ Self-Care/Independence	9, 16, 24

PSYCHOSOCIAL CARE SKILLS	
TOPIC	**QUESTION NUMBERS**
Emotional and Mental Health Needs	19, 47, 48, 49, 50, 51, 66
Spiritual and Cultural Needs	61, 62

ROLE OF THE NURSE AIDE	
TOPIC	**QUESTION NUMBERS**
Communication	30, 40, 53, 54, 55, 56, 57
Client Rights	31, 36, 58, 59, 67, 68, 69, 70
Legal and Ethical Behavior	63, 64, 65
Member of the Healthcare Team	60

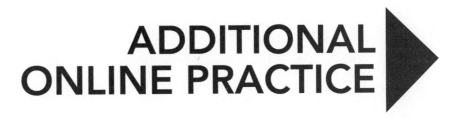

ADDITIONAL ONLINE PRACTICE

Whether you need help building basic skills or preparing for an exam, visit LearningExpress Practice Center! On this site, you can access additional practice materials. Using the code below, you'll be able to log in and take an additional one-time use, full-length Nursing Assistant/Nurse Aide practice exam. This online practice will also provide you with:

> **Immediate scoring**
> **Detailed answer explanations**
> **A customized diagnostic report that will assess your skills and focus your study**

Log into the LearningExpress Practice Center by using the URL: **www.learnatest.com/practice**

This is your Access Code: **8950**

Follow the steps online to redeem your access code. After you've used your access code to register with the site, you will be prompted to create a username and password. For easy reference, record them here:

Username: _____   Password: _____

If you have any questions or problems, please contact LearningExpress customer service at 1-800-295-9556 ext. 2, or e-mail us at **customerservice@learningexpressllc.com**